Kizzi's Health and Well-Being 2022

A revision of Your Well-Being Sorted! Originally published in 2014.

Research: James Miller, Helen Sykes, Melanie Jarvis-Vaughan, Peter Guthridge, Mark Gregory and Shawn Willis

Edited By Kizzi Nkwocha (c)

This edition is published with love and respect by Athena Publishing 2022

Kizzi's Health and Well-Being

All rights reserved. No part of this work may be reproduced or transmitted in any form or by any means, electronic or mechanical, including photocopying, recording, or by any information storage or retrieval system, without the prior written permission of the copyright owner and the publisher.

This book is presented solely for educational and entertainment purposes. The author and publisher are not offering it as legal, accounting, or other professional services advice. While best efforts have been used in preparing this book, the author and publisher make no representations or warranties of any kind and assume no liabilities of any kind with respect to the accuracy or completeness of the contents and specifically disclaim any implied warranties of merchantability or fitness of use for a particular purpose.

Neither the author nor the publisher shall be held liable or responsible to any person or entity with respect to any loss or incidental or consequential damages caused, or alleged to have been caused, directly or indirectly, by the information or programs contained herein. No warranty may be created or extended by sales representatives or written sales materials. Every company is different and the advice and strategies contained herein may not be suitable for your situation. You should always seek the services of a competent professional.

Kizzi's Health and Well-Being

Kizzi's Health and Well-Being is sponsored by Kizzi Magazine (www.kizzi.biz) and the relationship site MYVIP (www.myvip.me)

Also by Athena Publishing

Escape Your 9-5 And Do Something Amazing
Customer Service
SocMed: Social Media For Business
How To Start A Business With Little Or No Cash
Facebook For Business
Social Media Marketing: Write Up your Tweet
Getting Your Business LinkedIn
It's That Easy! Online Marketing 3.0
Business, Business, Business!
Mind Your Own Business
Insiders Know-how: Running A PR Agency
Energy Efficiency

Visit us at www.athenapublishing.com

Kizzi's Health and Well-Being

Well-being cannot exist just in your own head. Well-being is a combination of feeling good as well as actually having meaning, good relationships and accomplishment.
Martin Seligman

A grateful heart is a beginning of greatness. It is an expression of humility. It is a foundation for the development of such virtues as prayer, faith, courage, contentment, happiness, love, and well-being.
James E. Faust

The simplification of life is one of the steps to inner peace. A persistent simplification will create an inner and outer well-being that places harmony in one's life.
Peace Pilgrim

The well-being experts who contributed to this amazing book:

John Moore, Stina Garbis, Amber Asghar, Lulu Cook, Sylvia Tillmann, Sonja Courtis, Jamie Kerr, Jennifer McKenzie, Samantha Quemby, Robin Stoltman, Allison Jackson, Mark Newey, Rosemary Sherro, Julia Vearncombe, Amanda Price, Ciara Jean Roberts and Jo Hodson.

Gems Inside

Introduction	*14*
About Kizzi Magazine	*17*
Making A Deep Spiritual Connection in Your Relationship	*21*
Manifesting Love	*35*
Mindfulness and Meditation for the Curious	*46*
Mindset And Your Programming	*64*
Too Much Tension and Stress In Your Body? Shake It Off	*74*
When Our Beliefs Determine Our Well-Being	*85*
How To Become Successful In Business: Through Self-Love And Self-Confidence	*104*
The Power of Your Emotions for Physical and Mental Wellbeing	*121*
Building Resiliency Through Meditation, Mindfulness, and Mindset	*130*
Mental Wellbeing in Today's Digital World	*142*
Understanding The Mind-Body Connection And Our Emotions	*151*
Changing The Conversation On Mental Health	*165*
Meditation and Well-Being	*182*

Skin Confidence	*200*
How To Live A Long, Happy And Healthy Life	*216*
Healing Yourself	*232*
Beyond The Body: Journey of a Plant-Based Diet	*245*

Introduction

Welcome to Kizzi's Health and Well-Being. Our team of researchers and contributing authors have laboured for the best part of a year to produce a worthy update to our best-selling book, Your Well-Being Sorted! And this is it. Finally we can say those magic words: Welcome to Kizzi's Health and Well-Being. As a 2022 revision of our earlier title, Kizzi's Health and Well-Being offers new chapters, new topics and a wealth of information that will (I hope) prove invaluable in getting your pursuit of health and well-being on the right track.

For many of us well-being is not merely the absence of disease or illness. It is a complex combination of a person's physical, mental, emotional and social health factors. Well-being is linked to how you feel about yourself and your life. And yet, although we accept that well-being is important, it does, however, appear to be a little hard to come by. While researching Your Well-Being we came across a recent Australian consumer study into well-being that showed that:

- 58 per cent wish they could spend more time on improving their health and well-being.
- 79 per cent of parents with children aged less than 18 years of age wish they could spend more time on improving their health and well-being.
- 83 per cent are prepared to pay more money for products or services that enhance their feelings of well-being.

In our increasingly consumer-driven society money is often linked to well-being. The reasoning here is that having enough money should, theoretically at least, improve living conditions and increase social status. However, the reality is that happiness may increase with income but only to a point.

The fact is that wealth is not a fast track to happiness. Various international studies have shown that it is the quality of our personal relationships (with others and with ourselves), not the size of our bank balance, which has the greatest effect on our state of well-being. Indeed, believing that money is the key to happiness can actually harm a person's well-being. For example, a person who chooses to work a lot of overtime misses out on time with family, friends and leisure pursuits.

Today, with an astounding number of reports about increasing obesity rates, diseases and conditions related to being overweight and out-of-shape, it is impossible to ignore the importance of fitness and well-being in our lives. Health professionals attribute cancer, diabetes and mental issues such as depression to deficiencies in fitness and well-being.

However, it is often only when we are sick, injured, or the quality of our life is under threat, that we truly recognise the importance of health and well-being as we face up to the potential loss of well-being, mobility, or life itself.

As the publisher of Kizzi Magazine, Business Game Changer and My VIP I am often confronted by the irony that we devote more attention to the health and well-being of our family, our friends and even distant communities, than to our own health. That is what makes us human – our altruism and fallibility.

Many of us make choices about the way we live our lives that potentially damage our bodies or our minds – healthy choices are not always easy choices. For some, the 'lottery of life' delivers special challenges to health and well-being and living with a disability, chronic disease or disadvantage can be a hard reality. While concentrating on exercise and diet can help people suffering from disease and illness, one consistent thread running through this book is the belief that you shouldn't wait until you develop an illness to begin a health and fitness routine.

Kizzi's Health and Well-Being gathers the collective experience and knowledge of well-being practitioners from all over the world in order to offer you a guide to a much better life. With thought provoking and insightful chapters on almost every aspect of natural health, alternative and complementary medicine, Kizzi's Health and Well-Being is a valuable first step to a healthier, happier you. Enjoy.

Kizzi Nkwocha, Publisher, Kizzi Magazine, MYVIP, Business Game Changer, Middle East Game Changer, The UK Newspaper, The Property Investor and Money and Finance Magazine.

About Kizzi Magazine

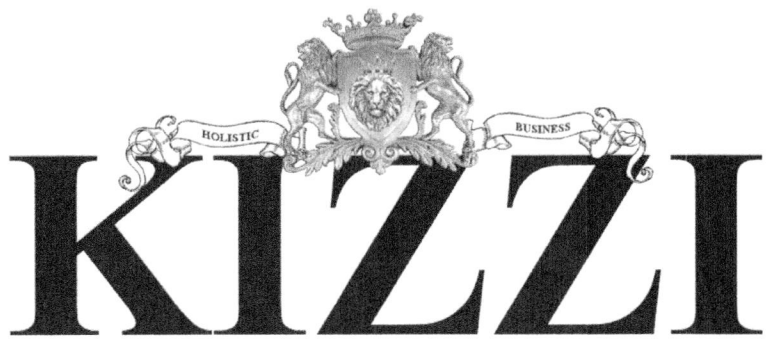

Kizzi Magazine is the world's only business magazine focused on holistic business strategies. Our editorial focus is on providing readers with insight on the psychology of business success while also maintaining the balance between profitability, wellness and corporate social responsibility.

The traditional business model focuses on physical input and output to drive results with little consideration for the other key aspects such as the wellbeing of employers and employees and anyone who comes into contact with the business, such as customers, investors, vendors, etc., also known as stakeholders.

Having a holistic approach to business means looking at business as a whole interconnected entity; understanding the bigger picture, not only thinking outside the box but removing the box completely.

The holistic approach to wellbeing has been around since the 4th Century BC, taught by Hippocrates who encouraged people to look at themselves as a whole person rather than just focusing on a specific body part or illness. Kizzi Magazine's goal is to bring this holistic approach to business. Developing holistic views on markets, businesses, companies, and products increase the likelihood of success and growth.

To many this is similar to a 'conscious capitalism' perspective in that a business is intentionally making decisions and taking actions to benefit all stakeholders.

Our thought-provoking features explore the healthy mindset and psychology required to manage a successful business, as well as the very practical and hands on steps you need to take in order to win in business. We are a progressive publication, with a distinct editorial focus on mindset and wellbeing within business as well as the practical issues of start-up finance, law, operations and strategy. Our community of writers also provide novel insights into the business founder ecosystem and the people in it.

Kizzi Magazine is a 4 'I's publication: Inspire. Inform. Influence. Innovate.

Follow Kizzi on Twitter: https://twitter.com/kizzinkwocha

Kizzi's Health and Well-Being

YOUR WELL-BEING AND RELATIONSHIPS

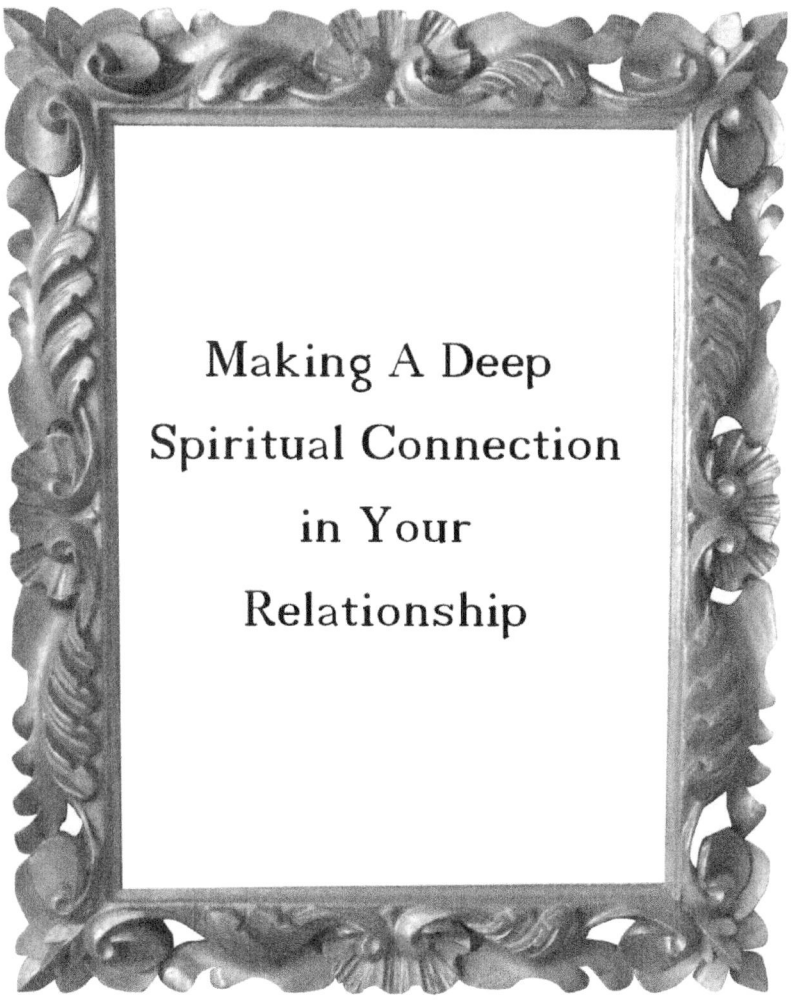

Making A Deep Spiritual Connection in Your Relationship

Making A Deep Spiritual Connection in Your Relationship

Love is a beautiful thing. It can be fun and exciting, but it also has the power to change you in wonderful ways. When you find someone who gets you, they inspire growth. They show you what's possible when two people come together on an equal playing field with their best selves at the forefront of every interaction. Forming a deep spiritual connection with your partner can not only make your relationship more fulfilling, but it helps both of you become your best selves.

People are complicated. To simplify, we have a body, mind, and spirit. Great relationships address all parts of us. Good relationships address our physical needs for intimacy and safety. They stimulate our thoughts and create loving emotions. Indeed, fulfilling relationships always includes the spiritual aspect of the couple.

Why would you want to concern yourself with the spiritual aspect of your relationship? Relationships that include a deep spiritual connection have many benefits. The relationship itself can become stronger on both a physical and emotional level. Each person in a spiritually connected relationship feels supported to live their best lives. As a couple, your resilience and ability to overcome difficulties increase.

Right now, you may wonder what I mean by the word spiritual. Does this mean religious? Do we need to practice the same religion? Do both of us need to meditate together? No, none of that is necessary. While it's okay if you have a spiritual belief system in common, I want to expand the definition of spirituality to be more inclusive.

My definition of spirituality includes religious, those who aren't, and even those who consider themselves non-believers. Spirituality is anything that makes us feel connected to something greater than ourselves. For you, that might be God, the universe, nature, the world, or anything. Spirituality includes connecting to your relationship and your partner profoundly and healthily. This definition of spirituality leaves room for anyone to reap the benefits of spiritual connection.

I believe that the deeper you go into anything, the more spiritual it becomes. Watch anybody who dedicates themself to pursuits such as a sport, or music, or art. There is a moment when they become completely absorbed into what they're doing. They step into a state of flow, and there is a connection that defies description.

I was talking to my partner about this recently. She said that she didn't like to watch basketball, but she would watch Michael Jordan play with the Chicago Bulls. If you watch someone of the caliber of Michael Jordan perform what they are passionate about, there are moments when they become absorbed. They enter flow with the universe in the same way someone does who is in deep meditation.

I can remember as a boy seeing a fantastic concert pianist play with a grand passion. His performance moved me emotionally. About halfway into the concert, I realized his eyes were closed despite his precision playing. It was almost as if the music were playing for him. It was a spiritual experience, despite no religious overtones, dogma, holy books, or clergy. This pianist was "plugged into" spirit, expressing itself as music.

Every human being can experience and express spirit like this but in their way. Relationships are dynamic, like basketball games and concerts. When you connect with your partner, you can express the same flow inside your relationship. You can have beautiful, transcendent experiences that strengthen your bond and help you through the challenges all relationships face.

As a teacher of shamanism, I act as a guide for my students to discover their spirits. Our spirits often express themselves through archetypal impulses. For example, in nearly every shamanic culture, the impulse to become a shaman is a response to a personal crisis. Not everybody feels a calling to a shamanic awakening, however.

Ancient mystics recognized that every living thing has two archetypal impulses. They called these impulses the divine masculine and the divine feminine. Though they used gender language, all people have both instincts no matter their sex or gender.

Modern philosopher Ken Wilbur named the divine masculine Eros and the divine feminine Agape after two Greek terms associated with love. The divine masculine, or Eros, represents the impulse to evolve. Growth and development exist in the very biology of everything living. Every living thing is subject to evolutionary forces.

Beyond biological growth, we have all experienced the drive to learn and develop. If you think back to when you were a child, you may remember things where you felt the strongest urge to learn—tying your shoe, riding a bicycle, learning to drive. I have a joyful memory of my daughter's determination to learn how to whistle when she was four years old. She told me, "Daddy, I will not stop until I can whistle, and then I will not stop whistling."

The divine feminine, or Agape, is the impulse to connect, network, and grow within a collective. Biologically, our cells gather to form organs; our organs form systems, systems make up our bodies. Socially, we connect with family members, friends, community, country, and world.

Despite what we see on the news, Stephen Pinker points out in his book, *Better Angels of our Nature*, that we are in the least violent era in human history. Indeed, humanity has a lot more progress to make, but we are coming together more and more. This impulse to care for one another expresses the divine feminine.

Within a profoundly spiritual romantic relationship, both partners feel supported in expressing both impulses. They can care for each other, the relationship, and others around them. They both grow as individuals in ways that might not be possible if not for the connection. The relationship is synergistic, meaning that the sum is greater than the individual parts. In extension, deep relationships have a positive effect on the world around them.

Prerequisites for having a deep spiritual connection in your relationship

How do you know if you're in a spiritually connected relationship? It worries me when I see people rush to label partners, soulmates, or twin flames. Sometimes this happens in very unhealthy codependent relationships. Many people confuse dependence with connection.

There are some essential preconditions for forming a spiritual connection with your partner. The deep relationship is healthy for both parties. There is no room for mental or physical abuse of any kind. Partners should be partners, meaning there's a power imbalance in the relationship. Communication and honesty are at the forefront of interaction, and both partners' feelings are equally important. The relationship elevates each person with no room for controlling or jealous behavior.

Almost every romantic relationship begins with powerful, positive feelings. This is wonderful, but a lot of this emotion results from hormones like oxytocin and parts of our brain wired for social connection. Who hasn't been in a relationship that started with fireworks but then fizzled as time went on? While it's lovely to enjoy the "honeymoon period" of a new relationship, you'll have to put effort into turning that into a fulfilling lifelong relationship.

Spiritual connection with a romantic partner takes time and effort. It isn't instantaneous. Michael Jordan wasn't born to play basketball. He worked hard for years. Concert pianists don't just sit down at a piano without a single lesson and crank out Rachmaninoff. However, there are certain qualities in a relationship that facilitate connection.

Vulnerability is a positive quality that includes sharing things about yourself that would otherwise make you uncomfortable. In a deeply connected relationship, both partners feel safe being vulnerable. Partners can share their most vulnerable parts without fear of shame or judgment. Each also feels free to be themselves with their partner. This safety can be a powerful healing force in the relationship. It may take some time before each partner feels safe enough to be truly vulnerable, but this is something you can each consciously practice.

In a deeply connected relationship, partners have and respect healthy boundaries. Good relationships do not consume anybody's individuality. Healthy boundaries can be rigid or flexible but always reflect a person's values. Each person should feel comfortable expressing and discussing boundaries around sex, finances, respect, expectations, etc. Partners should not use boundaries simply as a method of controlling each other's behavior. Accidental boundary crossings occur. It's a good idea for partners to check in with each other regularly.

When partners fully support each other, each person has the freedom and confidence to grow into their best self. Each person is free to find and follow their true path. This support is the divine feminine allowing growth, the divine masculine, to occur.

Why focus on having a deep spiritual connection?

Deeper relationships are fulfilling on all levels—physical, mental, emotional, and spiritual. A spiritually connected partnership provides the support and grounding for a life well lived on all fronts.

When you have a deep connection with your partner, your relationship will be a source of joy. With that joy comes better mental and physical health. Studies have shown that happy, positive romantic, and platonic relationships lead to healthier and longer lives.

Your relationships can serve as a "home base," making you more resilient to the natural difficulties of life. You have a sense of safety, a place where stress drops away, and someone on whom you can always depend. When you have this safety net, you can make better decisions in the face of obstacles. All parts of your life benefit,

Spiritually connected relationships can heal old wounds. Most people have had a variety of relationships, both healthy and unhealthy. Some of us experience trauma at the hands of a parent or a lover. Trauma and shame leave wounds in our psyche—shamans call these wounds soul loss. When you and your partner provide absolute safety from trauma and inside the relationship, there is room for healing the psyche.

Methods to connect in your relationship

Now that you understand some benefits of having a spiritual connection with your partner, I'd like to give you some concrete ways of creating that connection. Deeping a relationship in this way takes effort, but I hope you understand it will be worth it. I hope you will always consider your relationship a work in progress that can just get better and better, with no end to joy and love.

The fastest way towards any desire is to get into congruence. Congruence has the body, mind, and spirit all working together, moving in the same direction. To use an automotive term—firing on all cylinders. If I sit around wishing I could lose a few pounds while eating an entire chocolate cake every day, I am not in congruence and am unlikely to shed weight.

Likewise, if your goal is to enjoy a deep, joyous, and fulfilling romance, you'll want to get body, mind, and spirit working together. Below, I have given some concrete practices and suggestions. You do not have to do all of them at the same time. Try things out, see what works best for you, use them to explore making your relationship sizzle with passion and joy.

Body

When we think of physical intimacy, it's natural to think about sex. Humans are sexual creatures. There is no shortage of instructional manuals and spiritual texts outlining sexual practice. I would like to focus on some non-sexual ways of creating intimacy. I will draw from some Tantric teachings.

The first practice is eye gazing. Eye gazing is a simple but potent practice that can draw two people deeply together. In its simplest form, you sit facing your partner and merely gaze into their eyes. This is not a staring contest; you want to gaze and do your best to open yourselves up gently. It may surprise you at the intensity of this experience. You can try it for a few minutes at a time. During this practice, you remain silent and open.

During the practice of eye gazing, emotions may naturally arise. This is fine, let them. If you feel like crying, cry. If you want to laugh, laugh. The stuck emotional energy will come up. The feelings may peak, but they will subside. Allowing your emotions to move through you like this is healing.

To deepen eye gazing, sit very close–knees touching. Place your right hand on your partner's heart. Your partner places their right hand on your heart. You put your left hand over your partner's hand, and they do the same. The electrical energy field the heart gives off is hundreds of times stronger than the one given off by the brain. When people are connecting like this, their heart rates synchronize. Two hearts can beat as one.

After you have practiced eye gazing a few times with hands on hearts, there is an additional practice to create even greater physical intimacy. Add breath synchronization. Since you look gently into each other's eyes, use peripheral vision or touch to pace your partner's breath. As you both start breathing at the same rate, you will lose a sense of adjusting your breathing. You will just naturally breathe with your partner.

The following physical practice uses touch and communication to deepen intimacy. It isn't foreplay or sex but positive contact. The idea is to explore how you respond to different touches and practice listening to your partner's needs.

You can do this practice fully or partially clothed or nude if you're both comfortable. Once again, this is about non-sexual touch. You will take turns touching each other with one hand on different parts of the body, avoiding genitals or other erogenous zones. It's important to be gentle and to respond you your partner's feedback. If any touch is uncomfortable, you must stop it immediately.

As you take turns touching your partner, you gently ask for feedback. For example, you might place your hand on your partner's shoulder and ask, "how is that?" Your partner may respond with, "I like how that feels; it's warm. I think it might feel better, a little lower." Adjust based on feedback.

Mind and Emotion

The physical practices described previously will affect thoughts and feelings. Our bodies, minds, and spirits are overlapping and interdependent systems. The following methods are for the mental and emotional components of a relationship. These certainly can cause physical sensations as well, but the difference is the focus.

Empathy is one of the greatest gifts you can give to another person, and it costs absolutely nothing. Some people seem to have natural emotional intelligence that makes them empathetic, but it never hurts to practice.

It's easy to practice empathy and, when you do, the love between you and your partner will grow. You practice empathy by regularly imagining what it is like to be in the other person's shoes. Empathy differs from sympathy—which is just feeling bad for someone when things go wrong. Empathy creates an emotional understanding. We always appreciate it when someone makes their best effort to understand us.

Along with empathy goes non-judgment. Non-judgment doesn't mean that you allow your partner to ignore your boundaries or violate your trust. Non-judgment means that you may dislike their behavior, but you do not judge the person.

Another great way to connect emotionally is by expressing gratitude. Many consider regular expressions of genuine appreciation a "love language." Everybody wants to feel appreciated. Sincere gratitude will further endear you to your partner and draw you even closer.

Expressing gratitude is also great for a grateful person. Research shows that more grateful people are healthier and may even live years longer. The benefits to mental and physical health are significant and well documented.

Next is vulnerability. When both partners can share all parts of themselves, it shows trust. Vulnerability means letting down your defenses and letting your partner in, sharing your genuine feelings. When you trust your partner enough to be vulnerable with them, you naturally grow closer. Vulnerability also builds trust in the relationship.

Being vulnerable can help you work through your emotions. It allows you to relax and be your true self, increasing self-esteem and reducing stress. Your willingness to be vulnerable with your partner also opens you up for growth.

Vulnerability may be an area where you and your partner need to work. You can take small steps towards letting down your defenses. It helps to express your true feelings to your partner and let them know when something makes you feel vulnerable. Naturally, there has to be a sense of safety and trust in the relationship before partners can feel okay letting down their guard.

One of the most powerful gifts you can give another person is holding space for them. Holding space means listening intently to another without trying to fix them or offer advice. It allows the person you are holding space for to feel heard. I cannot overstate the positive effect this simple practice has on someone.

As a shamanic practitioner, holding space is a crucial healing tool I employ with clients. As a practice, it places them at the center of my attention. They can feel how important they are and that I am very interested in what they say. When your partner talks to you, hold space by listening to understand and not to respond.

To practice holding space, pretend there is a spotlight on your partner when talking to you. Listen intently. There is nothing more important at that moment than giving them your full attention. If your partner is complaining about something, ask them if they want advice or just want you to listen. When your partner expresses hard feelings, this is the time to practice empathy.

Spirit

Spiritually, it is essential to express your divine, masculine and feminine impulses and support your partner in doing the same. Support is the key concept here. You and your partner can and should work consciously towards a supportive relationship. When you do, the relationship will feel closer. You will each feel more freedom in expressing who you are.

How can you support your partner in expressing their divine masculine impulse? You'll remember that this impulse is the impulse to evolve, learn, and grow as an individual. Be your partner's biggest cheerleader. Support your partner in any endeavor to better themselves. Celebrate their successes while supporting them when things don't go their way.

Words of judgment-free encouragement go far. To be compatible, you do not need to have the same interests as your partner, but you can still support their passions. You should not try to direct your partner's self-growth. Doing so risks trying to change your partner for your interests. Instead, give your partner the space and support to find and express their true selves.

Your relationship can also grow and strengthen as an individual unit. Talk about and be open to the relationship developing. This doesn't mean putting pressure on your partner to make the relationship move forward. Discuss ways you can meet each other's needs. Communicate preferences using empathy and understanding.

When you work on your emotional connection with your partner, this itself expresses the divine feminine. The practices already mentioned will go a long way towards a stronger, more fulfilling relationship. You can also have honest discussions with your partner about what makes each of you feel more loved, heard, and understood.

Your romantic relationship may be the most crucial in your life, but it shouldn't be your only relationship. It's a red flag when people stop connecting with friends and family outside the relationship. It's natural to spend a lot of time together at the beginning of a relationship as the emotions and attraction are strong. However, a healthy romantic relationship leaves room for friends and family. Codependent relationships are frequently insular.

When each partner has the trust and independence to maintain friendships and family ties, your relationship will grow richer. It is important to have varied relationships. You can encourage your partner to connect with friends and grow their network without taking away from the quality time you spend together.

While you support your partner in their outside friendships, nurture your social connections. When you spend some time apart from your partner, savor the time you spend together. Acting on your divine feminine impulses, you will bring more energy and more love to the relationship.

A committed romantic relationship is one of the essential components of your life. Nurturing that deep connection takes work, but the effort you put in will be worthwhile. When the relationship is strong, it will nurture you and help you give and receive more love.

By John Moore

About the author

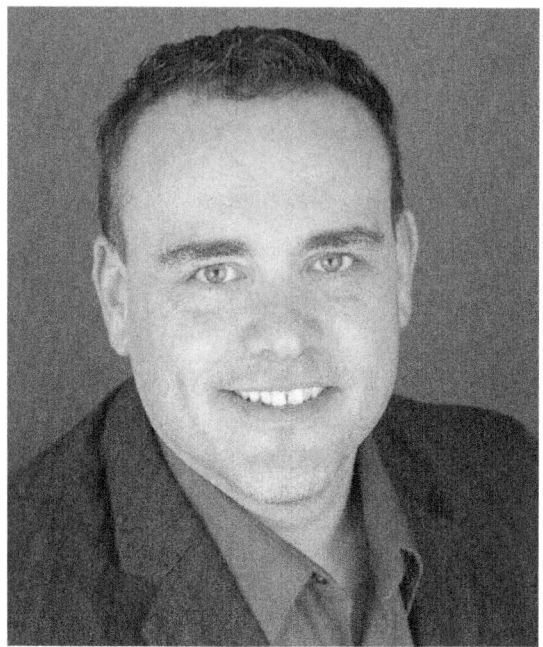

John Moore is a shamanic practitioner and teacher who works with spiritually conscious professionals to live fuller, happier lives, in touch with their true purpose. After two decades of working in the technology sector, John turned to humankind's oldest spiritual practice, shamanism, to heal himself.

John believes we interconnect with everything and everyone through a unique spark of divinity inside each person, making us co-creators of our reality.

John has written a column on the intersection of spirituality and men's health for The Good Men Project. He appears in a weekly radio spot, interpreting the dreams of listeners, and hosts his podcast.

John is a shamanic healer and teacher, having completed years of apprenticeship, advanced initiations, and shamanic teacher training. He holds a master's degree in Information Technology, an MBA, and a BA in Mass communication.

He is a 3rd-degree black belt in ketsugo jujutsu, a certified hypnotherapist, and a meditation instructor.

You can find more information about John at his website MaineShaman.com

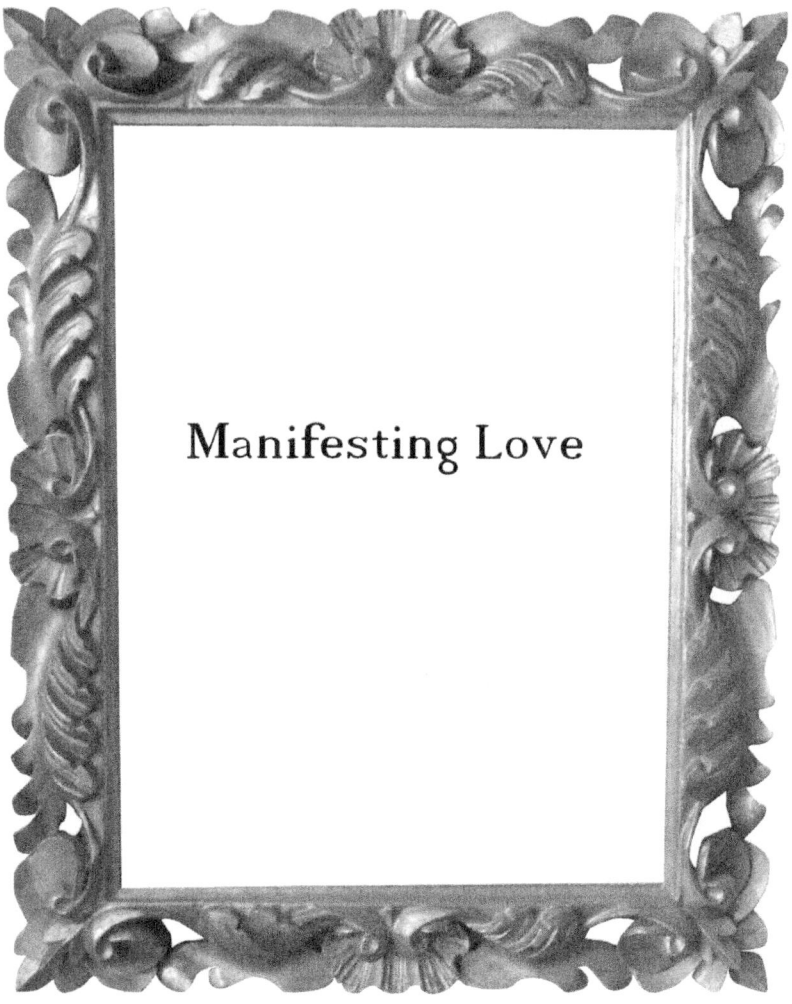

Manifesting Love

Manifesting Love

Our life up to now is made up of all of the decisions we have made, based on the thoughts in our mind. Our mind leads us into all of the scenarios that we have had and even affects us romantically. We act based on how we feel and our thoughts run those feelings. If we are feeling bad all the time and we are experiencing a lack of relationships or a string of negative relationships, it can be guaranteed that it all originated as a thought somewhere.

This thought sequence drives your relationship behavior. You can see it when trying to perceive your relationships. When you think of your love life, are you more blah about it, thinking "it's never going to work out" or "there's no good people out there" or "all people want to do is hook up"? We all have excuses like, "they never stick around" or "they never commit". Think about it right now if you are single. What is your excuse for your lack of love? It's okay to have one because inside of our excuses and our love life failures, exists a key to a better next time.

You may want to write some things down or use a section of a personal journal for some of these exercises. I'd like to go on a journey of what you want. It may be cliché to say that you can have anything that you want, but it may be more correct, that you can have anything you think about a lot. I've looked at my failing love life before and exclaimed, "Why"? Not understanding that a lot of what I was getting in my love life was what I was intentionally seeking through my negative attitudes.

Another way to put the Law of Attraction is to call it the Law of Expectation. What you expect to find is what you'll be aware of and then you'll see it everywhere. If you are proclaiming that there are no more fish in the sea and that the rest are rotten, then you can expect to find a bunch of rotten fish and you may run around with a rotten fish attitude. You may be repelling every available catch to you, that you may not even be aware of.

It is proven that all sorts of people can get into relationships. You can see it at the grocery store and at fast food places, love takes all shapes and forms. You don't have to be anyone special to fall in love or to have anyone fall in love with you, but you do have to be more willing to go along with then go against. We attract what we are in harmony with. Ask yourself is your mind in an at peace, loving, friendly and sensual vibration that is receptive to the giving and receiving of attention? I believe with smiling more and using times of mental adjustment and gratitude, we can attract some pretty great people.

This chapter is about manifesting your ideal partner, someone that you are in harmony with today. You don't need to wait to be perfect, because your mate isn't perfect either. You will catch them in their stage of becoming, as we all are constantly becoming more of who we are. There are certain laws that you can follow to attract anything you want and practicing "right thought" is one of those laws. There is a certain way to think, and when you want to attract anything, you must believe the truth, that love and abundance are everywhere at all times. People come and go in our lives and nothing stays negative forever. The first idea is to believe, and know from the bottom of your heart, that love is ever present and is available to you everywhere. There is no such thing as a lack of love, if you go into the world with kindness to yourself and others you will see love reflected back to you often.

To manifest romantic love into your life, you must form a clear picture of the desire of the love you want, and then use your imagination to draw this love into your life. Expect it to appear. When you truly desire something, you set up an invisible line between you and this idea. You can't desire something that doesn't exist, and when you strengthen your bond to the idea by fixing your mind on it daily, you are getting in harmony with it and it is being drawn into your life.

We attract who we are in harmony with, so if you are trying to attract someone above your pay grade or who has a dramatically different lifestyle than you, you may have a hard time. However, the person you attract may be on their way to that pay grade and lifestyle, just as you may be. You meet them where you are.

The first exercise is to determine where you are, and where you would like to go. Are you a working single mother trying to become financially independent, by owning your own business? Are you a student looking for your next step? Are you a powerful executive searching for an equal?

Write down a few sentences of where you are in life currently, because you will find someone with a harmonious situation, who may also be trying to get to the next step.

Write down a few sentences of where you envision yourself going in the next few years. These goals may be similar to the person you attract.

Next, let's look at what you are attracting. What if all of your relationships have ended in drama, or the people you are with are not reciprocal with their love? Are you attracted to what you want? Let's briefly brainstorm and affirm the opposite.

Write a list of characteristics that you attract and don't like. What do you complain about? Are they slow to respond or they never call back? Do they want sex without commitment, do they lack respect or are they pathological liars? We have all dated some characters. Write down a list of the problems you have been having in your relationships.

Look at your list. Do you see any trends? Why are you attracting these people into your life? Are any of these problems things that you provoke? What are your attitudes in your relationship? Are you going with the flow or are your expectations running wild? Let's begin to gently affirm the opposite and send love towards a different idea, and while you're at it send a little love to yourself and towards your exes and kiss them goodbye.

Write the opposites of your list. These are the things that you deeply long for in a relationship. It may be commitment and loyalty and respect. While you are writing your opposites, imagine, what does that look like in a partner? Don't put a face or name or form to this person or guess how they will come. Leave the miracle to the universe. But do start imagining what a loving committed partner feels like in your life.

Next, add to your list of opposites, what else do you want in a partner? Have fun with this and really dream of someone dreamy. Are they tall, good looking, funny and responsible? Do you want to share similar hobbies and interests? Would you prefer them to dress a certain way or be from a particular family background? What about religion, morals and how they treat their friends and family. What is their attitude towards life and daily living? Begin to imagine what a partner that is in harmony with you looks like. Add as much to your list as possible but remember, don't name them, give them a form, or guess the scenario where you will meet.

This list represents what you want in a partner, but may include some personal aspirations as well. Not only is this list someone you are attracted to, this person is attracted to you as well. If you are looking for fine qualities you need to match those qualities, by living your best, most kind, life.

Think about your list often, but remember, your person will be flawed and they need you to become even more of who they are. You are going to meet your person somewhere on the road to becoming great, maybe even at the beginning. When getting into relationships with people, they are always at a stage of change. They may have just moved, graduated, gotten out of a relationship and now they are meeting you, and both of your lives shift. Look back where you wrote where you are today. Your person will be in harmony with that. Consider, what does someone with good goals look like? What does someone with a direction look like? Can you also move in that direction?

The person you meet will be seeking you. However, the only way to set up this attraction is if you are seeking them with the same energy by being receptive to people around you, and by preparing for their coming. Get your house ready for company, make space for a visitor, get dressed as if you are about to meet someone that you want to impress.

Do things that promote social activities, join a discord, go to a paint and wine class, hang out with single friends and find out what they do.

Now that you have a clear picture of the type of person you want to attract, hang on to this idea as you are depositing it into the mind of the universe, or whatever else you want to call it. Start imagining that you are with them all the time. You are no longer alone in your mind. Take this person with you throughout your day, tell them everything, ask them anything. Say good morning, goodnight and amen with them. Using your imagination to be in constant connection with your ideal, it will manifest quickly, especially if you follow it with action by putting yourself out there. You can create a shopping list, but nothing is going to happen until you go to the store and pay your bill.

Taking an attitude of availability is necessary to attract someone great, but putting yourself on the market is what's going to help you manifest the one. How can someone buy a house when it's not for sale or there are no listings? First you need to be found where people are looking.

People invest money, time and effort into their careers and find success. What if you channel some of that energy and resources towards your love life? I sincerely believe if you are a single person, having an online dating profile is as important as having a savings account.

If you are worried about your identity or about the quality of matches, consider paying for a profile on a trusted site where people are verified and everyone is paying. That gives you a level of privacy and a possibility of more sincere matches because they are throwing money towards their love life which shows that they are more serious.

However, people find love on free platforms as well, where you may find a larger pool of people. Not everyone is going to be as nice on a bigger, wilder playground, but there are tons of opportunities for love there. I would say to choose what suits you but somehow show the world that you are available.

If you want to do anything well, you must research it and try to understand it. Look for how to put together a positive dating profile, by looking for examples online or enlisting the help of some savvy friends who are dying to see you get hitched. Don't throw anything up on the internet expecting great returns. Put some thought into it.

One tip is to not use overly sexy pictures. Try going for a friendly, person next-door vibe as it is less intimidating than being super sexy and unattainable. Always put a call to action at the end of your profile, telling your potential date to reach out to you. I like asking my new suitors to send me a clean joke to break the ice.

Remember, the goal of a dating profile is to get you an introduction, not a relationship, so keep it light. You don't want to come off sounding desperate for a serious relationship or express high expectations by listing a set of qualifications and rules that your date has to follow. Keep it friendly and open and slightly mysterious. You don't have to air your laundry online. Not everyone you meet will be husband or wife material instantly, but you should consider giving different types of people chances. You may be surprised that the person you meet is completely different from what you are used to, because you are getting in harmony with a higher ideal and the quality of people in your life may change.

It's possible that after all the effort you went through to put up a dating profile, you end up meeting someone, somewhere else, and that's okay. Dating online is signaling the universe, saying that you are willing to be available and do the work by meeting prospective partners and making new friends. This open attitude will radiate throughout your life and you may find yourself attracting more people in different situations during your day.

Realistically, it's probable that things won't work out with everyone. That's all part of dating and the process, but you still have to try and invest in your happiness. We meet people and experience our life lessons, and then grow together or grow apart. Each relationship is important because it is getting us to the next step. Be grateful for mini successes, and bless rejection, trust that you will soon meet the right person who will be in your life for a while. Spending deliberate time in the morning or evening writing down how you are happy that this person is in your life is essential. Be grateful and craft an affirmation like, "I am grateful for love in my life that is in harmony with who I am and what I desire." You may want to charge a crystal or a piece of jewelry with your affirmation and keep it on you as a reminder of what you are bringing into focus. Try writing your love affirmation for 60 days and see if your attitude changes and you become more receptive to the love that is around you.

Using the power of the mind, gratitude and faith, you can attract anything you desire. You were not destined to be unhappy. The universe wants you to be your best self and have everything you need to accomplish your purpose. When you focus on going in the right direction, and are willing to think in a certain way - that love is everywhere and for you, it's just a matter of time before you find love.

By Stina Garbis

About the author

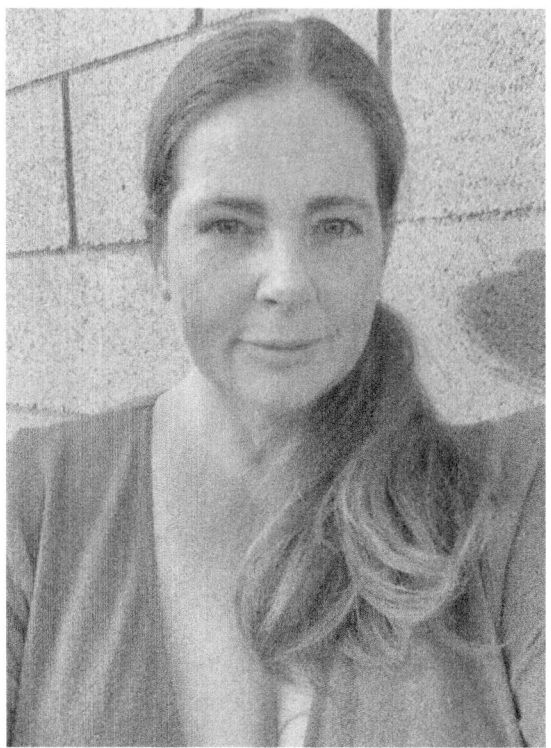

Stina Garbis is a professional astrologer and psychic and has been in practice for 30 years. She is @psychicstina on TikTok and Instagram. Follow for daily readings. She is the author of the workbook, "Find Freedom from Love Anxiety and Manifest an Ideal Love" available at psychicstina.com. Visit her website for more information or to schedule a private consultation.

Kizzi's Health and Well-Being

YOUR WELL-BEING AND MINDFULNESS

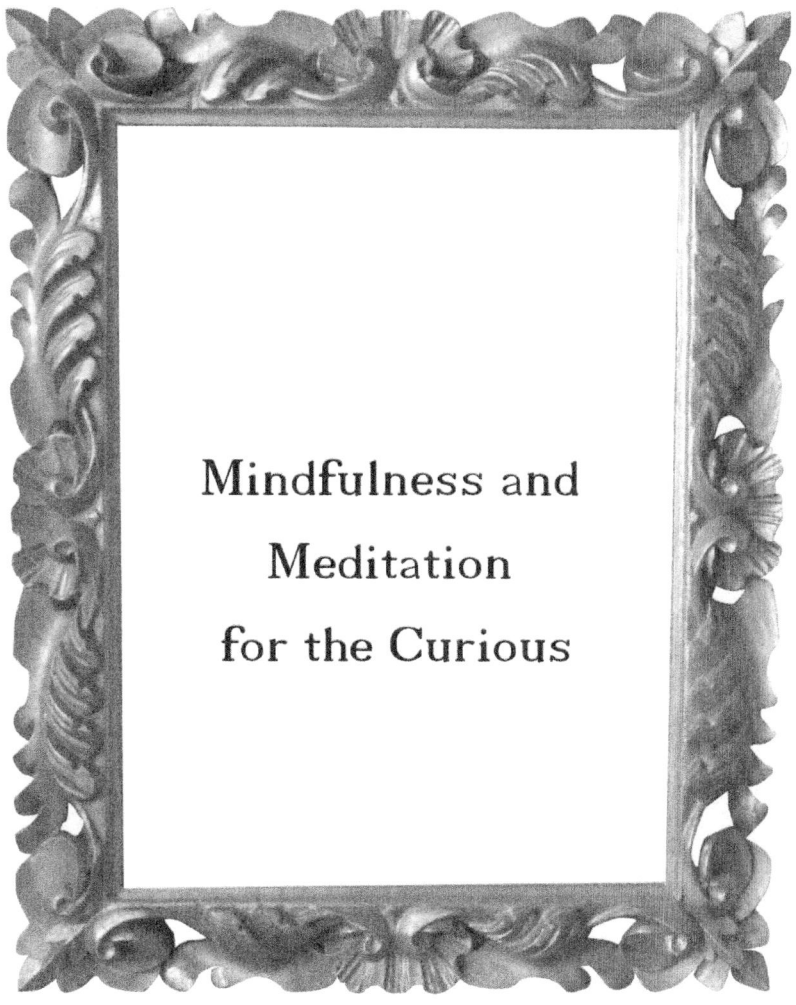

Mindfulness and Meditation for the Curious

Kizzi's Health and Well-Being

Mindfulness and Meditation for the Curious

What should I know about mindfulness and meditation?

Have you wondered whether mindfulness and meditation have something to offer you, but you're not sure where to begin, or what to believe about their effectiveness? Splashy headlines boast that these ancient techniques can cure everything from depression and anxiety to weight struggles and stress, all whilst enhancing your sense of serenity and happiness. These practices are effective at supporting well-being in many ways, but it's not always clear what the truth is, behind all the hype. In this chapter, we'll delve into the positive impacts mindfulness can have, and some of the many techniques to access the benefits. There are also common pitfalls that can derail attempts to cultivate mindfulness, and we'll investigate those as well. If you want to try it out, there are some simple exercises you can begin with, and tips for when you're ready to take your meditation practice further. There is no one right way to do it, and with so many options – there is a way to harness the benefits of mindfulness that will work for almost anybody!

First, let's define our terms. Every mindfulness program and research study out there seems to use a slightly different definition, but there is some general agreement that lets us make sense of it all. "Mindfulness" refers to intentionally directing attention to the experience of the present moment, while gently refraining from the typical mental chatter and judgements that often distract us. "Meditation" is one way to be mindful, often involving sitting still and choosing one thing to focus on, such as the sensations of breathing or a specific phrase.

You might think of mindfulness as an open awareness of what's going on in the present moment, while meditation focuses attention in a more concentrated way. With some overlap between these approaches and many different techniques for each, there is a wide range of ways for you to try it out and see what works best for you. Another term to be familiar with is "practice". This word is often used when discussing mindfulness, because these tools describe purposefully training, or practicing, to direct awareness in a specific way – not a final end goal. In this chapter, we'll talk about mindfulness generally, along with giving some specific ideas about ways to meditate, in case you want to try it out.

Why practice mindfulness? And why not?

Mindfulness practices are a natural complement to other activities as part of a positive and energized lifestyle. No single approach is the only answer to well-being – for instance, we don't only eat broccoli, and then call it a day with living a life that is healthy and vibrant! The true power of transformation comes when we weave multiple strands together, creating a tapestry of wellness that touches every aspect of our lives. Meditation and mindfulness are ideal supports for this approach, as we can bring this special kind of awareness to everything we do. This increases the momentum of our other well-being practices, such as physical activity, conscious relationships, work/life balance, financial health…there is no aspect of our experience that cannot benefit from the intentional awareness that mindfulness develops.

The research world is busy testing and documenting some of these powerful impacts as well. There were over 1000 scientific studies into the possible uses and benefits of mindfulness in 2015 alone, and the academic interest is not letting up. With so much research being pursued, there are bound to be conflicting results regarding where mindfulness helps, where it may cause harm, and even what, exactly, is being researched. This is not always obvious from the headlines, which often leave an over-enthusiastic impression that mindfulness can cure anything. While that's not the case (see the box below for some situations in which mindfulness should be approached with care), scientific reviews that consider the results of many different studies on the same topic suggest that mindfulness may indeed support some key areas of health and quality of life.

Consider with care: If you are at risk of schizophrenia, bipolar or other depression, post-traumatic stress disorder, acute substance abuse, or other mental health challenges, mindfulness practices should be discussed with your health care provider as part of an overall care plan. If you do decide to try it, look for an approach specifically tailored to the disorder you are addressing, and be sure it is taught by a trained professional.

Mindfulness has been shown in the science to help reduce anxiety, stress, and the recurrence of depression for some individuals. It may promote maintaining a good memory, whilst also helping with pain management. For those who struggle with harmful behaviors such as habitual alcohol use, mindfulness can be supportive in reducing or stopping consumption - perhaps because it helps people learn to tolerate cravings that arise and pass, without having to act on them.

Some meditation practitioners report other benefits, which may be harder to measure in a lab. For instance, increased awareness of our internal experience helps some people experience more presence and clarity in their lives. You may have heard someone talk about an increased sense of calm, gratitude, and emotional balance due to meditation, or you may even have experienced these yourself as you cultivate mindfulness.

However, expecting meditation to fix our problems, make us more calm, or improve our moods may lead to disappointment. When we bring our attention to what we are really feeling or thinking, it's not always so serene and cheerful! When we read those exuberant headlines about the latest study, we need to take into consideration our own experience, while using the actual science (not just the sound bite) to cautiously interpret claims we hear. Sleep quality, eating habits, and weight control are other situations where some people experience improvement when they incorporate mindfulness, while others may not. There is nothing wrong with whatever your experience is – that's one of the key things to keep in mind as you begin your journey. Mindfulness is an experiment, an investigation into getting to know yourself better, and it's best conducted with a sense of curiosity and friendly self-compassion for whatever comes up in the process.

What could possibly go wrong? Pitfalls and tips to get started.

Curiosity and gentleness come in handy, as it's common to face challenges in beginning and sustaining a mindfulness practice. Let's look a bit deeper into typical bumps that can arise, and some strategies for addressing them.

- **Make it a date.** Have you ever felt really motivated to try something healthful...and then just...forgot to do it? It is not uncommon for new meditators to get to the end of the day without thinking about meditating for a single minute! Our positive intentions can easily get swept away by the hectic busy-ness of daily life. Remind yourself that you don't have to jump right into meditating for an hour a day. Carving out just 5 minutes to bring awareness to your breathing or body can be very centering in the midst of daily stress. You might schedule your practice time in your diary or online calendar to prioritize it, or find a meditation buddy with whom you have accountability for following through on your healthy new habit.
- **Counter self-judgement with self-compassion.** Many people experience negative self-judgements and shame as a familiar internal refrain. These thoughts can be all the louder when you intentionally try to quiet your mind and focus on present-moment awareness. Self-judgement can come up before, during, and after mindfulness practice. If you've ever thought, "I can't do this, I'm doing this all wrong, I'm never going to get any better at this," during meditation, you've experienced this kind of negative self-talk. Learning to recognize these thoughts without having to believe them is one of the benefits some people experience with mindfulness. When the shame refrain arises, counter harsh self-judgements with self-compassion. Try saying silently to yourself something like, "It's hard when these judging thoughts arise, but I don't have to believe them. I can choose to be friendly to myself and continue with my practice".
- Adjust your expectations. Mindfulness is not a quick fix. It may take a long time before you feel more calm or begin to notice the benefits of practice in the rest of your life. Identifying any expectations about what mindfulness "should be" like leaves less room for disappointment, and more opportunity for you to practice from a curious, open-minded perspective. These expectations may occur while you are actually meditating, when thoughts arise that the session "should be" different than it is. Remind yourself that you are simply practicing present-moment

awareness, letting go of striving to somehow "get it right". Training your mind in this way is a big change from how you usually use your attention, so patience is called for.

- **Bring your body with you.** Many people find that they spend most of their time living "from the neck up". Our culture expects and rewards high function from a performance perspective...but that can come at the expense of experiencing our bodies in lively and vibrant ways. We may have even been taught that our bodies are unacceptable, or to disregard the wisdom of our bodies as irrelevant or lesser than things we "know" with our heads. This unfortunate divide means we are less present for the whole experience of our lives and cut-off from more intuitive ways of knowing. Body-based mindfulness techniques can help us return to kind awareness of our bodies. They help us tune into our "gut feelings", and access the information and guidance based in the rich terrain of our bodies, not just our brains. Try the Body Scan Meditation at the end of this chapter to begin to tap into the wisdom of your body.

- **Turn grousing into gratitude.** If mindfulness practice is just another thing on your list of things to do, it can be hard to feel motivated about it. Reframe your perspective by cultivating mindful gratitude as your practice. This can be as easy as taking a few deep breaths when things are getting crazy, and bringing to mind one thing you feel grateful for. It could take the form of a "Gratitude Circle" with friends– it can be very uplifting and grounding to hear from fellow members, listing a few things that they are thankful for via text or Facebook. If that's not your style, try writing in your journal each day, reflecting on the things you are grateful for and how you feel when you contemplate them. Giving yourself permission to make gratitude your mindfulness commitment can help transform just another "thing to do" into an energizing practice that brings a sparkle of awareness and joy to every day!

"Yeah, but..." What to do with excuses during meditation.
You may be thinking, "this all sounds good, but I actually do want to try meditating, and I just keep running into the same old issues!" Here are some of the most common excuses, and ways to work with them.

- **I can't stand the silence**. We are surrounded by noise and distraction in almost every aspect of our lives. We move from the sounds of the morning news show...to the ever-present beeping of electronic gadgets and ringing of cell phones...accompanied by an ongoing stream of commentary, opinion, and judgement carried on in our heads. It can be a confronting experience to turn all the machines off, and sit down with an intention to meditate quietly. The silence may seem to be drowned out by the uncomfortable roar of our own minds! One way to work with external noise is to intentionally try sound meditation, in which the noises all around us, and the sense-based experience of hearing, are what we bring our attention back to when we get swept away by thinking. When the uproar is coming from our own minds, we can bring our awareness to all that chatter, without necessarily believing any of it. You might also experiment with an approach called "labeling" in the box on the following page.

Work with it: A technique called "labeling" can help when we notice we've lost awareness of our meditation object (e.g. breath or sound) due to internal "noise". We apply a short label to the thought stream, then return our attention to our breath. Experiment with using the simple label "thinking", or be a bit more specific, labeling the thoughts as "planning", "remembering", or "wanting", for instance, before returning to your intended focus. The goal is to find a few short, simple labels that help you acknowledge those noisy thoughts, then set them aside. The mind is made to generate thoughts, so all that mental chatter is normal – yet we can train the mind to become less noisy over time during our meditation sessions.

- **I can't stay still.** Does it ever seem like the instant you sit down with the intention to be still, you begin to itch and feel uncomfortable in new and excruciating ways? Just because we have an intention to focus our attention doesn't mean our deep-seated habits of distracted multi-tasking disappear! If this is a challenge for you, it may be useful to prepare for meditation by engaging in light physical activity, such as going for a walk or doing a few minutes of simple stretching. This can help you feel relaxed and comfortable in your body when you sit. Find tips in the box on the next page for making mindful movement a primary practice.

Work with it: Some people choose to make mindful movement a primary part of their practice, or even their main way of practicing. Activities such as yoga, swimming, and tai chi invite participants to set aside their worries for a while and let their attention be fully present in the gentle movements and breathing that are key aspects of these exercises. There are even classes available for mindful running! There is no single "best" kind of movement, as long as you enjoy it and find it supportive of mindfulness.

Another approach is to make the impulse to move part of your awareness practice. Observe what happens in your mind when you commit to be still for several minutes, noticing what the desire to wriggle or itch feels like. Sometimes, bringing attention to how strong that urge can be is enough to release it, and you'll be able to return to your breath. Other times, you may decide to reposition yourself with mindful attention to each movement, and curiosity about whether it actually solves the problem of feeling restless. If you are truly in pain, then it's always ok to move - the following box gives guidance for working with physical pain.

Consider with care: Never continue with a meditation posture if it causes you physical pain. It is not necessary to sit on the floor, or cross-legged, or in any position that strains your body. It's hard enough to courageously face the truth of your own heart and mind, without adding in real physical pain from a posture that is not right for your body! If you are having a difficult time finding a sitting position that is comfortable and sustainable for you, or if you are experiencing pain caused by chronic medical conditions, consider working with a meditation teacher for guidance.

- **I just fall asleep every time I try to meditate.** It's common to struggle with sleepiness during practice sessions, and the solution may surprise you. It just might be to go ahead and take a nice nap! Many of us try to manage hectic, time-poor lives and jam-packed diaries by sacrificing adequate sleep. These habits can catch up with us as soon as we slow down to practice mindfulness. If you're in a particularly chaotic time in your life, you may benefit more from taking a little nap than from trying to meditate. Let your body get the rest it needs, then come back to try meditation again when your energy has rebounded a bit. You may find it much easier to stay alert and attentive then.

- **I've got the gimme's.** When we begin to practice mindfulness, we often notice that much of the meditation session is spent in wanting something. Whether it's yearning for a job or relationship to work out the way we want it to, fantasizing about the perfect holiday cruise, or wondering whether there's any ice cream left in the freezer, wanting is a primal response to the uncertainties of the world. And no matter how long we meditate, desire is not going to disappear for most of us. However, mindfulness practice can help us become aware of how strong that sense of craving is and how much of our time and energy it takes up. This awareness helps create more choice about whether we act on our desires or not. We work with craving by first acknowledging and accepting it as a normal part of our experience when it arises during meditation. We can bring curiosity to what yearning feels like in our bodies, and investigate any thoughts that go along with it, like a belief that "if only I could get X, everything would be all right" (see the box on the next page for more about beliefs). We learn to respond by noticing desire as part of our moment-by-moment experience, without beating ourselves up about it or getting swept away by it. Instead, we cultivate our ability to be aware and at ease with the present moment experience as it is. This creates real positive change in how we perceive the world.

Consider with care: Research shows that we experience something called a "hedonic treadmill", in which we believe we constantly have to acquire more of what we want in order to be happy. In reality, as we get or achieve more, our desires grow as well, so we need to top it next time in order to try to ensure our sense of happiness. Additionally, when we do get something we've dearly wanted, we may experience a short-lived increase in our perceived happiness levels, but this drops back down to our usual level of contentedness over time – this is referred to as an individual's "happiness set point". In other words, acquiring the thing we've been wanting does not ensure that we'll get and stay satisfied. Freedom from the tyranny of always wanting more comes through our willingness to sit quietly, noticing our experience and learning to be at ease with how things are in each present moment. Mindfulness actually helps us raise our own happiness set-point, no matter whether we get what we want or not!

- **I'm just so angry and irritated!** The flipside of desire can be feeling overwhelmed by aversion or anger. It can be frustrating and discouraging to feel surges of these intense emotions during our practice, when we hoped to enjoy an oasis of peaceful calm in our life. Yet it's normal to experience the arising of aversion or ill-will during meditation. Many of us have been taught from a young age that it's unacceptable to feel or express challenging emotions like anger. We may spend a lot of time and energy in daily life managing our emotions, projecting an attitude of cheery politeness, and "being nice". With so much effort exerted to maintain a pleasant front during the rest of our lives, meditation may be the only space we give ourselves to truly feel our feelings – including the difficult ones (see the box on the next page for tips on working with difficult emotions).

Mindfulness provides a powerful opportunity to get in touch with anger as a force that can drive beneficial change in our lives. These emotions can help us identify situations in our lives that are unacceptable or causing harm, and give us the energy we need to make difficult changes. Work with it: We can allow anger and aversion to be present, noticing what it's like to experience these emotions. We observe how our bodies feel and what happens in our minds when we are angry. The point is not to stoke any particular story that feeds the aversion, it's to allow the energy of it to be present and alive in our experience without trying to repress or manage it away. If you are experiencing anger or irritation in meditation, that's a perfect place to practice. If you are feeling overwhelmed by it, or not sure how to practice with it in a way that is helpful, consider reaching out to a meditation teacher who can provide guidance and support.

- **I'm distracted and doubtful.** Daily life can feel like a never-ending challenge that meditation could never help, yet it actually provides countless opportunities to practice mindfulness. Activities such as driving to the store or waiting in line can be so routine that we do them on autopilot, without even noticing. If anything happens to interrupt those routines, we may become impatient or even enraged almost instantly. For instance, think of the last time sometime cut you off in traffic –perhaps your heart pumped harder as you fought off an impulse to curse or tell the other driver to go drive over a cliff! These situations are "where the rubber meets the road" with our mindfulness.

When we learn to notice reactions and impulses that arise in us in response to typical daily irritations like these, we begin to build in a bigger cushion between the trigger (being cut off) and the reaction (yelling). We create less drama and wreckage in our lives, as we gain more ability to make thoughtful decisions about how to act when we are provoked. Ultimately, this leads to experiencing a greater sense of calm in parts of our lives that used to frustrate us.

Is there anything else I should try?
If you have enjoyed a positive impact from what you have tried so far, you may be ready to expand into new arenas. You may also still be looking for an approach that works for you. Either way, here are some additional things to consider.

- **Sample mindful eating.** Modern life makes it too easy to gobble down our food while at the desk, in the car, or in front of a screen. In these scenarios, we barely notice what we are eating, nor how it impacts our health. We can be so distracted, we don't even notice the tantalizing aroma and taste of our favorite dishes! Mindful eating reminds us check in with ourselves before we eat, noticing how our bodies feel and how hungry we are – or not. This encourages us to be more aware of the enjoyment we gain from the foods we consume, and it also helps us notice when we have eaten enough. Tactics such as putting the fork down between each bite and eating in settings without the typical distractions are helpful. When we commit to mindful eating, we build a few moments of present-moment awareness into our daily routine every time we sit down to have a nibble. It's a truly delicious way to practice!

- **Mindful in a minute.** Nobody needs to know we are doing anything special when we practice mindfulness. It can be as quick as taking a few deep breaths when we are feeling overwhelmed, to allow our attention to settle back into our body and the present moment. We can practice by simply bringing an attitude of curiosity and investigation to new situations we find ourselves in, such as moving into a new office or meeting someone for the first time. After we begin a regular practice of cultivating mindful awareness of each moment, we may find that we show up in these new situations differently. We develop more capacity to show up fully for what is actually happening with presence and an open mind. And nobody can even tell we are checking in with our awareness as we do so!

- **High tech mindfulness.** If harnessing the power of technology to develop your mindfulness practice sounds appealing, there are a wealth of apps out there to choose from. Some of these send text reminders to practice, provide timers and bells to keep track of how long you meditate, or provide guided meditations to follow. While different options come in and out of availability quickly in the app stores, a few well-known and long-standing apps to try include Insight Timer, Calm, and Headspace. If you'd like to practice mindfulness with the whole family, there are even apps that include the kids – for instance, you might try Smiling Mind.

What can I do next to deepen my practice?

Some people fall in love with meditation the first time they try it, or build up to that over time, and find they want to explore more. If you're feeling excited about mindfulness and you're ready to go deeper, here are some ways to develop your practice.

- **Sit more.** Adding a few minutes to your meditation every day can be a way to really go deeper. While there is no single, specific, or "correct" amount of time to aim for, many meditators find that sitting for 20 – 40 minutes each time allows their thinking to settle down and provides enough time to begin to experience a sense of calm. Others enjoy meditating twice a day, for instance 10 minutes in the morning and 10 minutes at night.
- **Find support.** A teacher or meditation community can be invaluable support while developing your meditation practice. A friendly, experienced teacher can answer your questions about mindfulness and give suggestions for ways to work with any challenges that come up. This does not have to be a mystical guru or a monastic recluse; there are plenty of "ordinary people" who have long and dedicated training in meditation and who can offer meaningful guidance in the areas of daily life that can seem difficult to bring mindfulness. Many people also discover a sense of quiet and steadiness that arises when they meditate with others. An internet search for "meditation" or "mindfulness" groups in your area will get you started. Be sure any groups you are considering are a good match for your values, and that the teacher has experience and training in leading meditation.
- **Go on retreat.** Silent meditation retreats can be like jet-fuel for your practice. Carving out anywhere from a weekend to ten days, or more, for mindfulness and meditation may seem like an impossibly huge commitment…and it can be the biggest gift you will ever give yourself. Retreats typically take place in a supported setting, with a teacher, other dedicated students, and no worries about daily logistics as meals are provided, and your cell phone will be turned off. While meditation retreats can be challenging (you're there with your own mind, after all!), they also offer giant rewards in terms of the clarity, wisdom, and compassion that can arise from concentrated practice. They can also be very motivating for continuing to practice when you return home.
- **Don't forget the heart.** There are meditations that intentionally cultivate the qualities of a tender and loving heart – practices such as compassion, forgiveness, gratitude, and kindness. Far from being just an "extra", or something to try after we achieve some other goal, these techniques are an integral part of practice from the very beginning. Consciously cultivating these qualities can be a powerful antidote to the

sense of isolation and disconnection many people live with, allowing us to connect more joyfully and lovingly with others. Additionally, many people find the heart practices to be a natural and easy way to access states of concentration and focus that may elude them with other meditation approaches. If you're curious to give it a go, you can begin by selecting a word such as "peace" or "love" to use as your meditation focus for a whole session. Continue repeating that word to yourself throughout the meditation time – and don't forget to apply it to yourself, when you notice your thoughts drifting away!

Your path to developing a sustainable and enjoyable practice of meditation and mindfulness will be unique to you, and there is no one right way to do it. As you learn to listen to your present-moment experience with friendliness, you may reap benefits such as the development of wisdom and kindness, increased presence for the fleeting and precious moments of your life, and increased ability to tolerate discomfort without acting out on it. You may learn new ways of working with physical pain and mental distress, or bring fresh awareness to other aspects of developing more healthful habits. However, the path to developing these gifts can be rocky at times. Our busy lives make it difficult to prioritize our own wellness in many ways, including meditation and mindfulness. Once we do carve out the time, it may be shocking and difficult to deeply listen to and feel the thoughts and emotions we often sweep aside.

The courage to persevere is already within you, and you can draw upon it to transform your own life with clarity and emotional steadiness. Be gentle with yourself as you begin to practice regularly. Don't beat yourself up. Try lots of different techniques, and give them some time. Find an approach that feels energizing and supportive and stick with it. There are great benefits to be uncovered, you are worth the effort, and you can do it!

Breath meditation instructions:

A simple way to practice meditation is to focus on the breath. Even well-seasoned meditators continue to use this method, as the breath is always present, yet every time we inhale and exhale, it is a new and different experience. As you prepare to try it, consider setting a timer for 2-5 minutes, so you won't be worried about how long you've been practicing. You might like to read these instructions out loud in a slow and steady voice and record them, to play back as guidance during your period of meditation. Begin in a comfortable posture. If you are sitting upright, let your back be straight and your hips and feet evenly balanced beneath you. It's fine to use a chair if that's comfortable. It's also ok to lay down, although you may be more likely to feel drowsy if you do so. Invite yourself to be alert yet relaxed as you begin. Remind yourself that there is no way to do this wrong, and that you are simply experimenting with becoming more mindful.

Start with three full, deep breaths in and out. Feel your lungs expand as you inhale fully. Enjoy the feeling of this deep breath, then let it out by exhaling slowly. Take your time inhaling and exhaling three times.

(Pause)

Bring to mind your intention to practice awareness of your breathing. Remind yourself that it's the mind's job to generate thoughts and feelings, but you don't need to get lost in them right now. When you become aware of having gotten distracted, you can set the thoughts gently aside until your period of meditation is over.

(Pause)

Allow your breath to return to a natural, steady pace. Observe where you feel the breath most strongly in your body – perhaps your nostrils, chest or belly. Wherever you sense the breath most strongly, place your attention there and notice what it feels like to breath in and out.

(Pause)

There is no need to force the breath to be a certain way. Simply notice whether the breath is fast or slow, shallow or deep. Observe each breath with curiosity, continuing to focus on the physical sensations of each breath.

(Pause)

If thoughts or feelings have distracted you, gently bring your attention back to the next breath. Inhale, and notice where the breath is strongest. Exhale, noticing the sensations of releasing the breath, and let the thoughts fall away.

(Pause)

Remind yourself of your intention to practice awareness of the breath in this meditation session. Whatever it was like for you was just right. Acknowledge your own efforts in training your attention in this new way.

Take another deep breath if you like, then open your eyes to end your meditation session.

Body scan instructions:

Cultivate awareness of your body with a body-based meditation practice like this. You might read these instructions out loud in a slow and steady voice and record them, to play back as guidance during your period of meditation. Body scans can take as much or as little time as you prefer, depending upon how long you have available. Begin in a comfortable posture. If you are sitting upright, let your back be straight and your hips and feet evenly balanced beneath you. It's fine to use a chair and it's also ok to lay down, although you may find yourself more likely to become drowsy if you to do so. Invite yourself to be alert yet relaxed as you begin. Remind yourself that there is no way to do this wrong, and that you are simply experimenting with becoming more present with the sensations of your body.

Start with three full, deep breaths in and out. Feel your lungs expand as you inhale fully. Enjoy the feeling of this deep breath, then let it out by exhaling gently. Let your belly and rise and fall with each breath. Take your time inhaling and exhaling three times.

(Pause)

Bring your awareness to your feet, noticing any feeling of pressure where they rest against the ground, or press into your legs. Let your attention travel up your calf, observing the sense of the gravity pulling you toward the ground. Notice any sensation in the area around the knees. Focus on your upper legs, where they contact the surface beneath you or where your hands rest on them. There may be areas that feel numb or lacking in sensation, and that's ok too. You're simply investigating, bringing curiosity to the experience of being in your body.

(Pause)

Now move your attention to your torso, noticing first the sensations of gravity where your body makes contact with the seat beneath you. Let your awareness move up into your belly area. We often hold tension here, so allow your belly to rise and fall with the next breath. Release any contraction in these muscles, and feel your belly loose and spacious. Remind yourself that it's ok to relax for these moments.

(Pause)

Let your awareness rise up, into the chest area. Take a breath, and observe any change in your heart rate. Let your attention pour down your arms to where your hands are resting, and note the sensations there – perhaps temperature, tension, or even your pulse can be felt. Now bring your focus to your back and shoulders, noticing any tension or pain. Invite yourself to relax in any areas that feel tight, knowing that you can't force relaxation to happen. You are simply opening the possibility that the muscles may melt and relax under the warmth of your gentle attention.

(Pause)

Let your awareness drift up through your throat, observing any sensations. Notice your face, inviting the muscles in your jaw to relax, inviting the muscles behind your eyes to relax. Let your curiosity travel to the back of your head – can you feel the back of your scalp? The very top of your head? Remind yourself that you are simply practicing becoming more aware of what's present in your body, what the actual sensations are in each moment.

(Pause)

If you noticed any strong emotions or thoughts come up during this practice, you may make a mental note to investigate them further, perhaps through journaling or another meditation session. Take a few deep breaths, inhaling and exhaling fully. Thank yourself for taking the time to get to know what your body is feeling in this moment as you open your eyes and end the formal meditation period.

By Lulu Cook

About the author

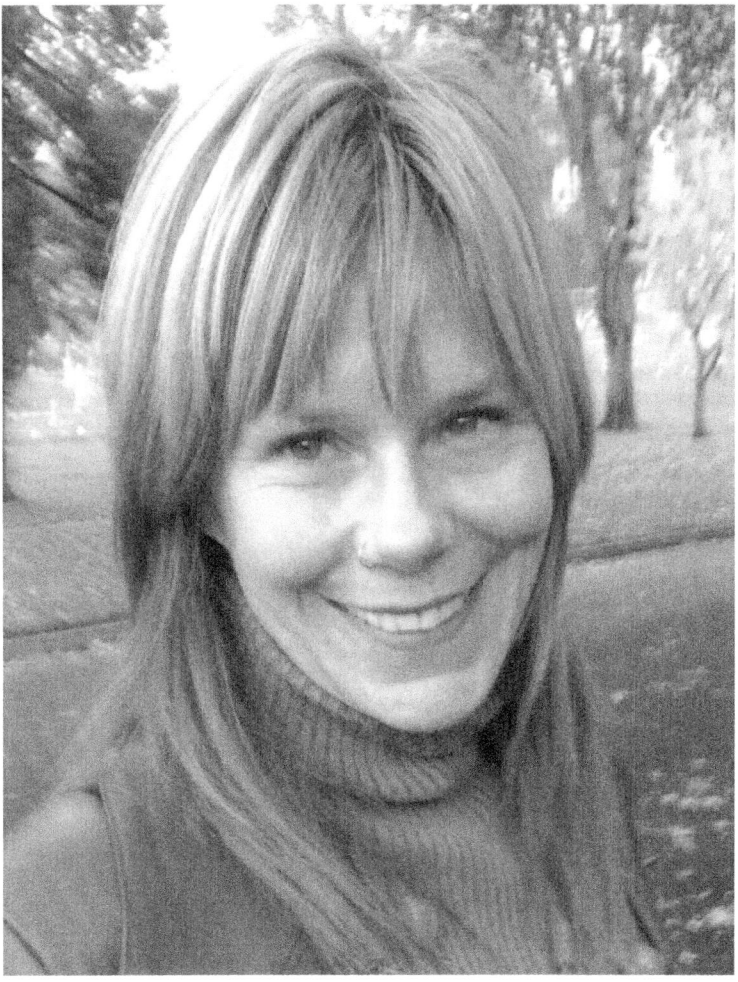

Lulu Cook, RDN, is a holistic health coach, author, and meditation teacher based in Brisbane, QLD.
She first began meditating in 2003, and began incorporating mindful eating as a nutritionist shortly thereafter. She has practiced in, studied, and taught at multiple meditation centers in the US and Australia since then.

She enjoys supporting students in initiating and sustaining a mindfulness practice, teaching mindfulness to teens, and addressing potential challenges that may arise for some meditators.

Lulu also has expertise in intuitive and mindful eating principles, which she applies in her Gut Feeling Holistic Health Coaching Model. She believes that each individual has an innate and trustworthy impulse for healing and balance that can be uncovered and enjoyed through body-based and other mindfulness practices. Lulu coaches from an integrated perspective that incorporates evidence-based and personalized nutrition strategies, and other wellness approaches in order to help clients experience sustainable, joyful elevation of their energy and health, and vibrant well-being in every facet of life.

Find out more at www.lulucook.com.

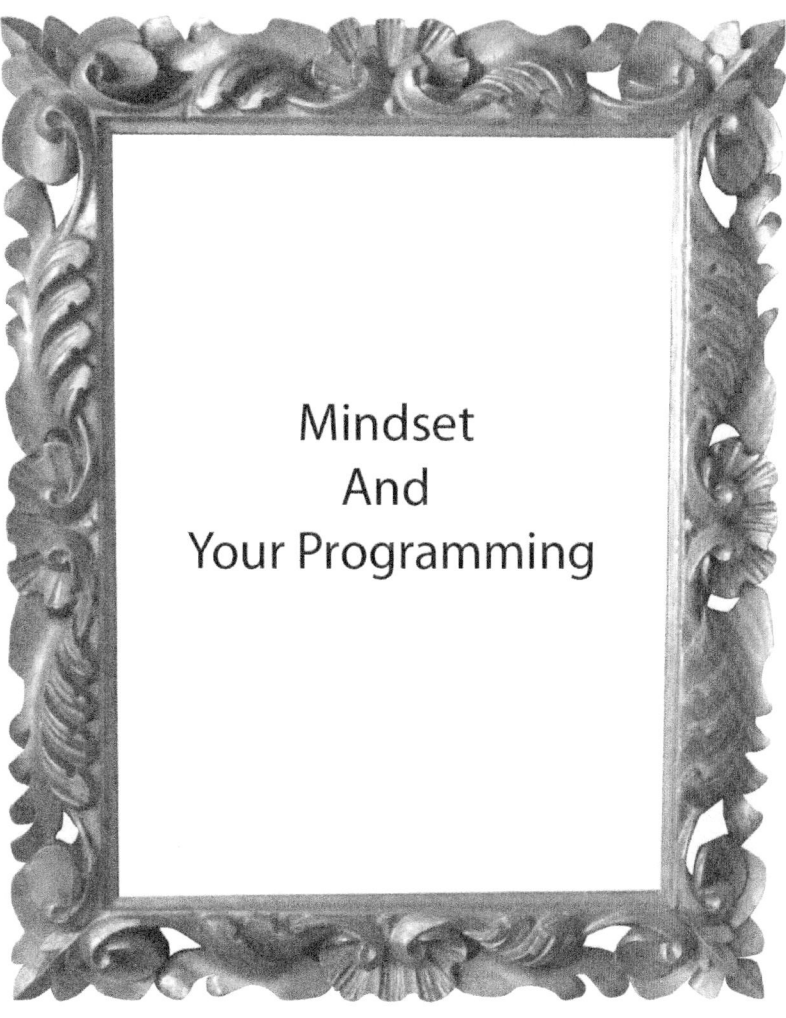

Mindset
And
Your Programming

Mindset And Your Programming

What does the term "mindset" encompass and how did you get your programming?

Everything in your mind that you cannot see. Why you do what you do in your life for habits, beliefs, values, morals, emotions, thoughts, imagination, intuition, long term memory, developmental stages, addictions, and how creative you are is all part of your subconscious mind.

Many people refer to the subconscious mind as your unconscious mind and or refer to it as auto-pilot as it's automatic behaviors, thoughts, emotions and everything above I just mentioned. These programs are running 95% of your daily life without you being aware and or conscious of the world around you.

As you were being formed in your mother's womb, anything and everything she took in, so did you. She ate beans for example you got the nutrition from those beans delivered via the umbilical cord. Your Mom took medication you got that as well via the umbilical cord. Your Mom experienced stress and so did you.

If your mom experienced joy, so did you. From the time of conception, you took in all this information as the absolute truth and as an experience of the world around you while you were developing. If your parents wanted a girl for example and instead, they got a boy they may have felt disappointment.

That disappointment you could have taken on energetically as shame. Which shame is feeling you are a mistake as you would be born feeling like a disappointment for not being the sex your parents wanted. The underlying root cause of disappointment is shame.

It does start this early in life for taking on someone else's feelings and choosing to make it your own feelings. This taking on someone else's feelings and or thoughts as your own is empathic behavior. This is how your emotions, traumas, and thoughts start being programmed along with the above I previously mentioned in general of what your mindset entails.

Being your programming starts at conception. You may be asking yourself then where do your beliefs come from? If you heard your parents yell or argue about money you learned what was said and the actions of how your parents treated money. You accepted this as truth. Many believe money is the root of all evil.

The truth is no it is not. Money has no value unless you choose to give it value in exchange for something you want. Money being evil is impossible as a hundred-dollar bill stays wherever it is placed until a human being picks it up and chooses how they are going to use it.

If a person has a bad intention towards using money for gambling or they may choose to give it to charity, this is an example of you viewing their programmed behavior along with your perception of how you chose to perceive their actions. It is not the money itself that is the actual problem in this example.
It is a positive intention either way for how the person chose to spend that money based on their programming they got as a child. This example goes for anything in life both good and bad as it all comes down to our programming.

Once you are born you are still learning about the world around you and how it functions. You put things in your mouth to learn if that object is food or a toy. You discovered how to use your legs to crawl then eventually how to stand to walk.

You took in information from the world around you using your sight, hearing, smell, taste and touch. Using this input known as data to help form more of your beliefs, and habits. This data serves you in your everyday adult life, so you do not need to keep relearning 'what is food?' versus 'what is not food?'

This is called generalization and it serves your brain in an efficient way, so you do not have to relearn something you come into contact with every time that you already know how to do or use. The subconscious mind stores this as known.

When you took in that information you also deleted things like the color of a toy you played with as that is not necessary for the brain to remember it. If you peed in your pants during the potty-training phase and were hit or spanked by your parents, you would remember not to do that behavior again as it was a disappointment to your parents. You could have internalized this as shame for being a mistake versus guilty of making a mistake.

This could also be a deletion of your parents working on teaching you to not to have accidents. This can make you choose not to trust them the next time you have an accident. So instead you may hide it - which leads to more shame of being a mistake. The deletion of certain things is to help your brain not be super overloaded as it truly does not need to remember every detail of your life in order to function.

This spanking can turn into a distortion of this event as to whether or not your parents love you or if they hate you based on the behaviors your parents consistently show you over time through consistency. Your subconscious mind will remember this love or hate for any possible future events proving either way the spanking was done in your mind out of love or hate.
All these examples I gave show how these events could affect you as a small child as they do affect you into adulthood. You cannot see your programming as this is how the subconscious mind operates to protect you and keep you alive at any and all costs.

Your subconscious mind also believes whatever you tell it as absolute truth well into adulthood. In fact, your time as a child for believing everything in the world around you - no matter who gave the information - forms many filters, with one being the reticular activating system.

These filters are fully formed by age eight. This means as an adult you can tell yourself all you want that you are a multi-millionaire. It won't happen if the world around you while growing up never gave any evidence you could see or feel with all your senses that it is possible for you to be a multi-millionaire prior to that age eight when those filters were formed.

Your subconscious mind checks these filters that were formed prior to age eight to see if this is a known or an unknown program for being a multimillionaire. If it is unknown - meaning the brain won't accept it as true due to lack of experience of feeling and being in the multi-millionaire mindset - the brain rejects, it and resists it thus preventing you from achieving the status of a multimillionaire.

The filters in your mind are to help guide and protect you. Being your subconscious mind is feelings-based running 95% of all your automatic behaviors, thoughts, emotions, etc, if your mind doesn't feel something to be true it based on what it knows it will come against these filters known as resistance. This prevents change from happening. This is why change is difficult to do on your own. In fact you are operating daily with only 5% of your daily awareness you have in life.

Your conscious mind is your logic, reasoning and will power that is formed after eight years of age. This is why sticking to a diet or what you would like to have happen doesn't happen without changing your mind's program at the subconscious level. The conscious and subconscious mind are not in full alignment.

Based on what I have already explained you cannot reach your goals in life or make any changes using your logic, reasoning and /or will power when you are only 5% consciously aware. Bearing in mind that 95% of your unseen or automatic programs come from your subconscious mind.

Can you change your beliefs, values, and or anything stored in your subconscious mind including trauma? Yes. You can. This is why hypnotherapy combined with neuro linguistic programming (NLP) is the most powerful tool for creating permanent change over any other method.

In fact, NLP and hypnosis is used in marketing of every product, or service anyone buys. Without it being used no one buys the products or services. I recommend reading, The Power of Habit, by Charles Duhigg, for more details. Or you can read, Copywriting Secrets, by: Jim Edwards, for more details even further of how marketing truly works when it is successful.

Both NLP and hypnosis I mentioned affect your subconscious mind and your conscious mind to have your goals become aligned. The NLP speaks to the nervous system of your body to create instant change. The hypnotherapy creates change by making something you want to be known in your subconscious, like being a multi-millionaire, easier to obtain regardless of your programming from childhood.

If your parents and society are against people who are rich, which most people are programmed into believing, you can use hypnosis to change your emotions, and thoughts to make it known that rich people are not bad. It is the intention of the person with the money that may not be so great via your perception from your programming. With hypnosis you can visualize or imagine yourself having the life you dream of as a multi-millionaire.

Many people refer to hypnosis as guided imagery, guided meditation, or meditation as it is more generally accepted by society. In fact, many coaches like life coaches sell you programs titling them as meditations when it is really hypnosis. Using these strategies that attract the goal you have closer to you as the subconscious mind is no longer going to resist you having more money is how the hypnotherapy (hypnosis, meditation, etc) combined with NLP works over any other methods out there.

You will not know on a conscious level why you are resistant to money for example. Your subconscious mind does know why. People who are trained professionals like me who have attended college for hypnotherapy know how to create that change you are seeking. I know many people believe they cannot be hypnotized and that is a lie from people who do not know what they are doing or who have had very little training.

Hypnosis is the state between awake and sleep. It is the dream-like state you go into every night and every morning. In fact, you cannot sleep without going into hypnosis first or wake without passing through hypnosis. This is why the last thirty minutes before you go to bed is super powerful to take in a new idea on your own when read out loud or written.

Handwriting is a direct link to your subconscious mind towards getting new beliefs, or habits for example you would like to have. It is the best time to stay away from anything negative like social media to prevent what you do not want to come into your life. Instead use this time to think positive happy thoughts both before you go to sleep and when waking up setting positive intentions for the day. This allows you over time to start finding more of the joy in life.

That joy raises your vibrational energy to attract more of what you want in life at a faster rate. This applies to money, relationships, children, etc as the mind will always give you more of whatever you choose to focus on - whether good or bad. That is how you can start to shift your life on your own until you make the decision you do want to change and have a qualified professional hypnotherapist who is also trained in NLP like myself help guide you to have that change even faster.

A few things you can do on your own is to read books like, Think & Grow Rich, by Napoleon Hill or The Science of Getting Rich, by Wallace B. Wattles. These books fully explain how powerful your emotions and thoughts are as you are constantly creating the world around you whether it's good or bad.

This is why it's true you are the average of the five people you are around the most including their paychecks. If you do not like something in your life you can always change it by seeking someone to help you get that change. You do have all the resources you will ever need in your own mind which is why when working on any goal it's best to start with the end in mind.

How does starting with the end in mind help you? Staying with my multi-millionaire example right now your reality around you does not reflect your vision of you being a multi-millionaire; what you would look like, feel like, act like, or be like. Start by writing down everything you see in your mind of what you view of yourself being and doing as a multi-millionaire. This is your end goal using this as your vision of what you want to read out loud or silently every morning and night of the person you are becoming.

This helps the mind focus more on bringing what you are seeking closer to you. In time it provides a clearer picture of what you are seeking as well in addition to a lot more details that you may not have previously thought of. This time can be considered true meditation as you are not listening to anyone talk via a recording of any kind.

You are simply focusing your time and energy on creating this new reality you wrote down you wish to see yourself as and having. You need to focus on feeling the experience of already being a multi-millionaire. When you do this as it will further help guide you to attracting it by raising your vibrational energy towards your goal.

Anytime your mind, and body feel content about having what you already are seeking, the body naturally relaxes and brings it to you in time. Before you do get what you want there is always a lot of internal resistance that rises, and it starts to show in your external outer world. That is the time to keep pushing through whatever happens by doing your best to stay positive and focused to still get what you want by keeping your end goal in mind. You can do anything you focus your mind on.

By Robin Stoltman

About the author

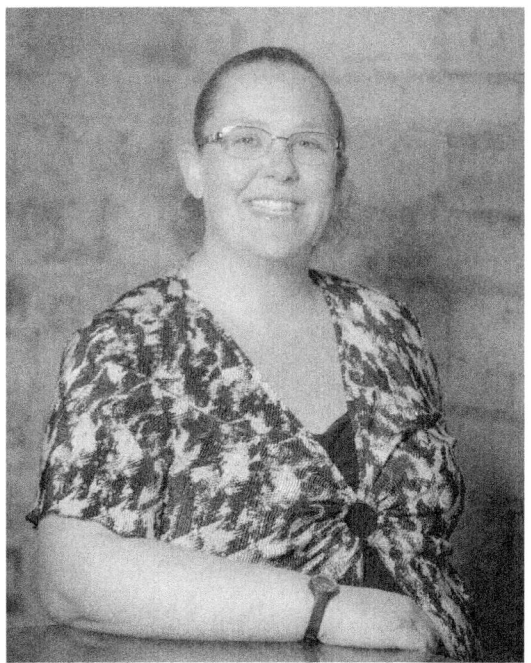

Robin Stoltman is America's #1 Intuitive Parenting Expert and Healer, Author, and Podcast Host. She is the founder and CEO of Healing for the Soul+ LLC. Her mission is to help Moms who have special needs children unlock the power of their own mind to have anything they want.

She was inspired to create her company after surviving multiple childhood traumas, a severe brain injury and then having Minnesota Child Protective Services steal her first son at just four days old without any court orders or proof. Now she helps people in releasing negative emotions, anxiety, and self-limiting beliefs related to all of life's challenges.

In addition to her diploma in Hypnotherapy, she is certified in over 20 areas related to the mind and body. Robin earned a director's award from the nation's only accredited college of hypnotherapy, Hypnosis Motivation Institute. She has been featured in over 12 media outlets such as Giddy Magazine, Authority Magazine, Thrive Global and many others. Robin is a statewide resource for mental health in South Dakota's 211 resource Helpline.

You can find her on social media under Robin Ann Stoltman, Robin Stoltman, or Healing for the Soul depending on the social media outlet you are using. Be sure to follow her podcast, Healing for the Soul Podcast via iTunes or on Amazon Music for more life changing topics.

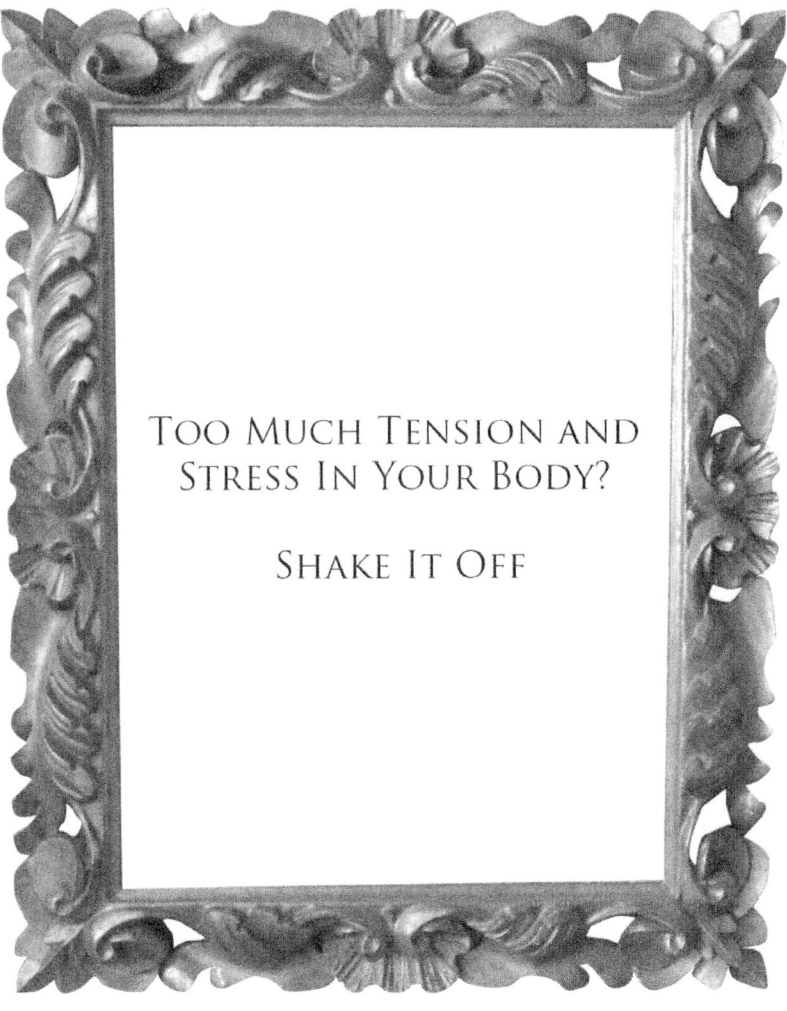

Too Much Tension and Stress In Your Body?

Shake It Off

Too Much Tension and Stress In Your Body? Shake It Off

What is more important – the mind or the body? No, that is not a trick question, I am genuinely interested in what you think. Does one score higher than the other or is it completely equal?

Maybe you think that the spirit is missing in this equation. Or you simply state that mind and body are intrinsically linked.

And yes, they certainly are, but I am wondering if we generally put too much emphasis on our minds, while ignoring the body?

Appreciating the mind-body connection is a fairly new concept in Western medicine – in contrary to Eastern medicine and philosophies that have always seen it as a unit.

In the Western world and in the 21st century, we want to talk things through when life is tough. We might even see a therapist to analyse the situation as we want to make sense of it all.

Do you also feel that you are much more in your mind than in your body? Many of us are obsessing over thoughts and are constantly overthinking, unable to stop the wheel and the endless thought processes.

Our minds are permanently switched on and busy with day-to-day thoughts, music or television in the background, the permanent stimulation by electronic gadgets, the ongoing multitasking and so on – why are we not giving our mind a break and engaging the body instead?

Welcome to the concept of somatic modalities

What does somatic mean? The Greek word 'soma' is referring to the physical body, hence the focus is on working with the body, rather than the mind. And this can work wonders for any psychological, not just physiological challenges.

There are many different somatic approaches, and you might have heard of practices like Tai Chi, Qi Gong, Alexander Technique, Feldenkrais Method®, EMDR, movement therapy, yoga, Pilates, Aikido to name the more well-known ones.

Let us first explore the benefits of body involvement, though. Even Sigmund Freud, the father of psychoanalysis, said all these years ago: "The mind has forgotten, the body has not – thankfully".

This sums it up perfectly in my opinion. Sometimes we just don't know what the root issue is, we might not even want to talk about it or are unable to cognitively verbalise anything.

Still, we might struggle with certain health challenges which your GP simply – and probably rightly – explains as "it's linked to stress or emotion" or "it is psychosomatic".

This diagnosis might be followed by prescription medication, maybe CBT (Cognitive Behavioural Therapy), counselling sessions or the simple advice to take it easy, to de-stress and relax.

That might sound like reasonable and well-intentioned advice, as the situation has been caused by stress, but how easy is it to *really* relax? And how can we effectively do it?

Stress and (not just big T) trauma

Let's take a step back and explore what is happening in our bodies when we experience a stressful, even traumatic event.

First I want to clarify, though, that "traumatic" does not necessarily mean big T trauma. On the contrary, it can include many events, that we might not immediately label as trauma.

Think of the fact that life itself starts in a traumatic way – the physical event of birth. And it is almost impossible to go through life without coming across some form of trauma – that is a part of life.

Dr Peter Levine, who has researched stress and trauma for 50 years, has been a stress consultant for NASA's Space Shuttle and who is the creator of another somatic modality, Somatic Experiencing®, explains it like this:

> "Trauma happens when the energy that we mobilise to defend and protect ourselves doesn't get used up. If we wanted to run or fight and couldn't, that energy gets stuck inside of us and as a result, many chemicals like adrenaline and cortisol get stuck, boosting up that energy and keeping it at that high level as though our survival energies are all dressed up with no place to go."*

Imagine our ancestors, who were out hunting or gathering and encountered a bear – their bodies supported them by producing the energy that enabled them to fight or flight. This is an amazingly clever and innate support mechanism.

Nowadays, there are – generally speaking – no wild animals that threaten us. Living in current times can still be stressful, but it doesn't necessarily cause us to run away or physically fight with the person we are having an argument with.

As a result of this inactivity, the excess energy doesn't get burned off and lingers in our system, which, over time, can get exhausting.

Levine explains: "This activation can stay on for years until the body is able to repeat the responses that it wanted to do at that time. And it doesn't matter what caused the stress or the trauma, what's most important is the completion of the response.

The effect of this undischarged energy is that we are on high alert all the time, and this can feel as if we are expecting, seeing and perceiving danger in many situations."*

You might have been around people who are permanently on high alert, they seem to be expecting danger and are scanning the room for threats – simply because their bodies are in constant fight or flight mode and their stress level baseline is raised. Quite often they are addicted to these very chemicals. Living under stress is like constantly living in survival mode.

As a result, one might also experience psychosomatic complaints, e.g. headaches, neck or shoulder pain, high blood pressure, sleep difficulties, gastrointestinal issues, anxiety and so on.
Or people might avoid scenarios that remind them of situations that caused the trauma, e.g. falling off a ladder as a child might turn into a fear of heights.
"The undischarged energy is what gives rise to symptoms of trauma, but this survival energy – that was there to prepare to defend ourselves – is waiting to be used up.
With appropriate guidance, this energy can be accessed and discharged at any time,"* states Peter Levine.
It is equally important to discharge the energy after freezing as endorphins are being released during the process and also need to leave the system, rather than staying trapped.

Let's get the body moving

Can you already see why I believe that somatic work can be so helpful? Read on to discover why it makes so much sense to include, rather than ignore the body.
As you have seen above, the excess energy can be discharged by movement, but, as you probably agree, we don't tend to employ motion as a stress response in modern society.
Bessel van der Kolk, the author of the best-selling book "The Body Keeps the Score" and himself a psychotherapist explained in a recent lecture:
"In order to deal with trauma, you have to work with the body. Trauma shows up in the body and it's important to ask: how can we feel safe and calm in our bodies?"**
He went on to admit that "psychotherapists only have a very small scope of what they can do for people and that maybe yoga teachers, bodyworkers, choral conductors, martial arts instructors and others may have at least as much to offer."**

As a somatic practitioner, I wholeheartedly agree. I would even go one step further by saying that once you have learned how to discharge the excess energy and the tension in your body, you can heal yourself without relying on anybody "to fix" you. You will have a tool to help yourself at any time – retrospectively or preventatively and for psychological as well as physiological pains.

Shaking is natural

So, let me introduce you to my favourite somatic process of releasing stress and tension. It is based on the fact that all mammals are genetically encoded to tremor in order to de-stress and it really is an innate reaction. David Berceli, PhD, observed that our bodies naturally want to shake to get rid of stress, but then our minds interfere and usually win. Unless it is an extreme situation, where we can quite often observe people who are trembling. Children do so, too, as they have not been socialised out of this process.
Berceli studied the body's natural reaction and compiled a novel way to support it. He put together a set of exercises to help the body to generate tremors.
He called it Tension and Trauma Releasing Exercises, TRE® for short. Berceli taught TRE® all over the world, especially to communities affected by war and conflict.
His participants reported good results with regards to PTSD (Post Traumatic Stress Disorder) – and Berceli formalised his method and created a training programme with certification.
TRE® is still a secret, even in the health and well-being world, so read on to discover how it can support your mind as well as your body.
What is your reaction when you see somebody shaking after a stressful incident? I guess the majority of us would try to comfort that person, try to calm them down and assure them that all is good or will be good soon.
Admittedly, a trembling body looks helpless, upset, maybe out of control, but this is simply based on our social and societal standards and the fact that we perceive tremors as weakness, embarrassment and possibly even illness.

However, shaking it off is so good for us as tremors enable a disrupted nervous system to bring body and mind back into balance. Berceli explains that tremors calm down the nervous system and complete the cycle, i.e. the excess stress hormones are being burned off as no longer needed.

Now you have a better understanding of what is happening in your body, you know what shaking can achieve and how it can help.

But what can you actively do to dissolve the excess stress hormones and release the tension you are holding in your body?

Let's get practical

Having completed the TRE® training and certification process, I teach my clients to help themselves. In fact, I empower my clients as – once learned – they can pro-actively support their health and well-being.

By eliminating tension, we can nip many stress-related ailments in the bud, e.g. tension headaches, migraines, back pain, teeth grinding, irritability etc. and help ourselves to become more resilient.

Let's explore this somatic modality in more detail. If you want, you can watch the official TRE® video on my website and can follow the instructions given.

Alternatively, many people want to experience TRE® for the first time with a trained Provider who can guide them, check in with them and simply be there to hold the space for them.

Both approaches are fine, but please don't dismiss TRE® as "it's not working" when you've only ever watched the video and practised on your own without guidance.

What can appear as quite an easy method is indeed a very powerful tool. As with everything else you are learning, it might be a good idea to lay the foundation with a qualified teacher to achieve the best results.

Either way, TRE® starts with six warm-up exercises that are similar to yoga stretches and aim to fatigue the muscles.

When teaching, I then guide my clients through a grounding exercise. This is important as I want my clients to feel safe and comfortable – and also open-minded and relaxed enough to explore the tremoring sensations with curiosity.

Lying on the back, we then move into the butterfly position, which means we put our feet sole to sole, the knees are automatically moving out and after lifting the body for another stretch, the actual TRE® process starts and the legs start to tremor.

Admittedly, it might sound strange and your mind might *think* "gosh, that's a bit weird, I am lying on my back, like a beetle and my body is tremoring!?" Probably, though, your body *feels* more like "wow, that is amazing, I have been waiting for this release for such a long time!"

Keep in mind that tremors are an innate mechanism to relax the muscles. This process is encoded in the DNA of mammals – and that includes us humans.

Trust your body's wisdom

The tremors are generated in the brainstem, the reptilian brain and its part that regulates unconscious reflexes and basic functions like heartbeat, breath and motor coordination. Although they are "just" appearing, you are in control and can stop the tremoring process at any time by stretching out your legs. This self-regulation is key in this tension-releasing approach, as proposed by TRE®.

When tremoring, the body releases chronic tension – that's basically all that's happening, but the knock-on effects you can achieve by having a more relaxed body and a re-booted and balanced nervous system can be immense.

As stress is the root of (almost) all evil, imagine how well you can support your health and well-being by clearing stress-related tension and therefore addressing psychological as well as physiological complaints.

Notice, I specifically said "stress-related". As tremendous as TRE® is, it's not a cure-all for everything, but it is most certainly possible to support your health and well-being with respect to tension overload.

The beauty of somatic work is that you stay in the present. It is a mindfulness practice and enables us to connect with our bodies again.

Do you sometimes become aware that you don't really feel your body anymore as you are living far too much in your thoughts and in your mind? Then it is my recommendation to get back into the body. Practising a somatic activity can help you focus on your body and its sensations.

In TRE® we don't verbalise any (past) events or analyse certain situations and it is quite liberating not to do so for a change.

Additionally, TRE® can also be a very helpful tool alongside cognitive therapies – especially when the client is stuck in the process. As a somatic modality, it can help to untangle the feeling of being stuck and move the topic of the talking therapy forward.

Although David Berceli developed TRE® as a self-help tool to support communities affected by war and conflict and has worked successfully with many PTSD sufferers, I want to re-emphasise, that TRE® is not just for people who have experienced big T trauma.

Living through the stresses of daily life – whether it is job or family related, or the pure fact that we have just lived through a global pandemic – is a good enough reason to pro-actively support your well-being.

Practised regularly, TRE® can dissolve the tension we are already holding in the body as well as preventatively combat stress and increase our resilience.

Learning from our dogs

If you are still not sure about the whole process, you might want to observe a dog after a stressful encounter – and you will find that the dog immediately shakes it off and then happily gets on with life.

Dog lovers have always stated that there is so much we can learn from our dogs, e.g. living in the moment, daily exercises, true loyalty etc. – let's add "shaking it off", too.

Isn't it time you'll give it a try?

Maybe that is still a question that shouldn't address your mind – so do ask your body instead. Your body most certainly knows.

Sylvia Tillmann

All quotes by Peter Levine, see Healing Trauma:
https://www.youtube.com/watch?v=PEf9KI4SWM8

Bessel van der Kolk's lecture on **https://www.pesi.com

_____

About the author

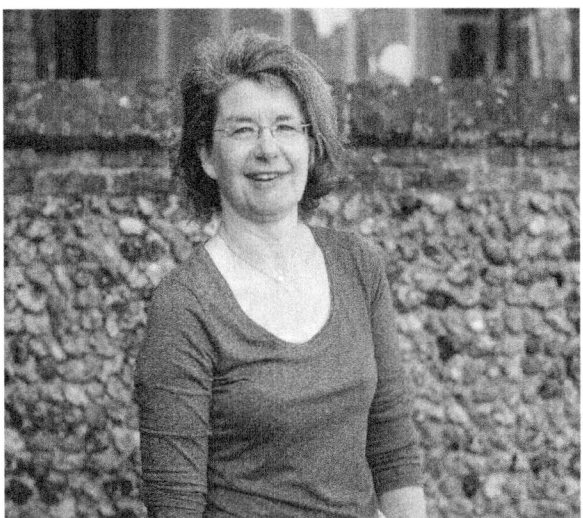

Sylvia Tillmann is a TRE® Provider and has a business and IT background. She knows very well what stress is. Although she used to dismiss it as "but I am having fun", its impacts were there: teeth-grinding and lower back pain.

Now she empowers her clients to take their health and well-being into their own hands, well bodies. She teaches how to – literally – shake off tension related aches and pains and states: "It is absolutely possible to feel better, become more resilient, empowered and even save money." Her teaching is informative, gentle and empathic and she has a foundation training in counselling (COSCA).

Sylvia truly believes that stress really is the root of (almost) all evil, but also knows that we can support our bodies to release stress and tension. She runs regular online courses, so get in touch for a free fact-finding consultation on www.tremendousTRE.co.u**k**

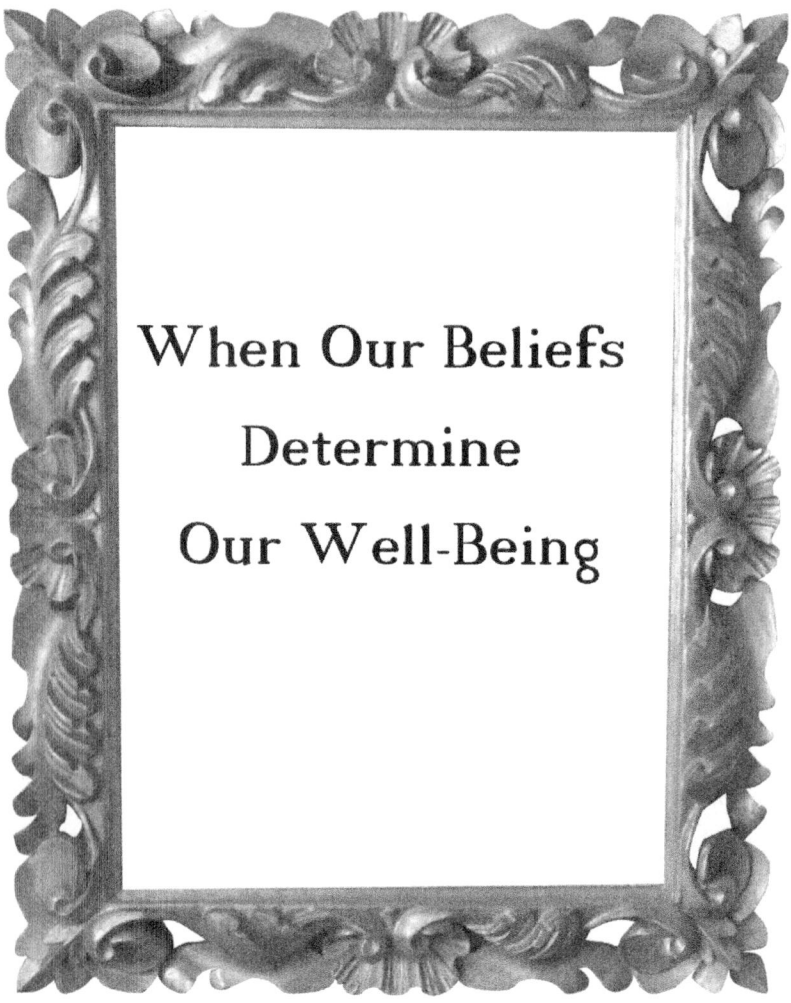

When Our Beliefs Determine Our Well-Being

Have you ever stopped to consider why, as a western society we are getting so sick? Why, with all the modern medicine and interventions are we not yet curing cancers and other illnesses? Why we are being afflicted with more and more supposedly new and incurable diseases? And lastly, why are more and more people turning to 'alternative' therapies to seek wellness and wellbeing?

When we think of 'wellbeing' the traditional approach is to consider the state of our physical body first, and address the issues there. Usual interventions such as western "allopathic methods" (the process of isolating symptoms and treating them individually with physical interventions such as specific medicines for each ailment) are the most common way we deal with illnesses and disease in western society.

If that doesn't work we are often left to believe we just need to live with said physical pain, illness or disease for the rest of our lives. Life becomes greatly shortened or lacking in quality when we are in left in this position of no hope and not knowing where to turn next.

This belief that there is nothing that can be done, is in itself harmful to our ability to heal because if they have not found a medication to treat the symptoms or a medicinal cure, then there is nothing that can be done to heal the physical body. And that rigid thinking has westerners dying in their 100,000s. This approach is reductionist in its thinking, as it isolates the physical issue and does not address the 'whole' picture causing the physical disease. It makes the assumption that diseases are stand alone separate physical occurrences with no links to our emotions or psychological wellbeing.

For the purpose of description, a disease is in fact 'dis-ease' of not only the body, but also the mind/emotions and the spirit. Allopathic methods see the body as separate from the mind and therefore it should be treated as such. However, scientific research now tells us that this is actually not the case.[1] So my intention for you in this chapter is to define well-being as I see it as a holistic practitioner, and provide examples of how people have achieved wellbeing through alternative Mind Body Spirit therapies. It is also my intention to provide insights into why we get sick in the first place and what you can do to get your well-being back.

I would firstly like to define 'healing' in terms of alternative medicine. Healing is the idea that the presenting physical issue is no longer having any evidence of physical symptoms in the body (in the absence of medication), and further to that, healing means we no longer have the associated emotional and mindset issues that also presented themselves prior to, and during, the illness and disease phase. Healing is of the mind, the body and in some cases, the spirit/soul.

Secondly I believe it is important to define 'well-being'. Well-being is not just feeling good in our physical body's, well-being is the absence of all illness, disease and pain symptoms and an overall general feeling of emotional and psychological happiness, contentment, inner peace and joy about ones life.

Well-being encompasses positive beliefs, optimism, enthusiasm, gratitude, hopefulness and a life lived in congruence and aligned to ones deepest desires and wishes. When I talk about well-being, I envisaged that there is a sense of overall satisfaction with life. There is the absence of chronic stress, anxiety, illness, disease, physical pain and any other issues of the psychology (mind) or physiology (body).

---

[1] www.ncbi.nlm.nih.gov/pmc/articles/PMC1456909/

"Alternative" approaches are becoming more mainstream and sought after and this in itself speaks volumes of peoples' realisation that more needs to be done to improve wellbeing than just taking medications. As a further definition, I will also be using words such as; complimentary, integrated and holistic, under this banner of 'alternative' treatments. Of course, we would be fickle to "throw the baby out with the bath water" so to speak in regards to ignoring western medical intervention, as they most definitely have their place and I believe it folly to ditch all western medicine altogether when looking at wellbeing. But evidence is mounting that we must not rely solely on allopathic medicine, there are integrated approaches that are needed[2]. Yet I know (from reading the research and seeing my own clients' results) that wellbeing requires a much deeper exploration than just the physical symptoms that appear. We need to peel back the layer on our inner workings, our emotions, our levels of stress and our mindset, environment and nutrition to really get to the bottom of why we are becoming so unwell. Particularly in western countries where we have seemingly huge advances in medical interventions yet we are not getting any healthier.

---

[2] Ester Sternberg MD, Andrew Weil MD

What I want to share with you today is the notion that, modifications to our diet and our physical wellbeing and lifestyle can only take us so far to true wellbeing. A healthy body is the start, however for this to occur, it has become even more important to have a healthy mind/emotions and spirituality. The latter two are the areas I specialize in in bringing about an overall sense of wellbeing for people (alongside their traditional interventions) and therefore by focusing on the emotions and mindset, physical well-being is even more likely and more possible (but more about that soon). We have insurmountable research and information available to us now that inform us how our emotions and mind are just as much responsible for our health and well-being as our diet, exercise and nutrition.[3] And it is at this point that I would like to introduce the concept of beliefs and how these impact our overall health and our own likelihood of being or becoming unwell. Fortunately, alternative approaches can heal these beliefs and bring about true well-being.

---

[3]Herbert Benson M.D, The Relaxation Response; Craig Hassed M.D, Monash University Medical School

Let me introduce you to Samantha*, a middle aged women with a list of physical issues as long as your arm; fibromyalgia (a joint inflammation illness of the autoimmune variety), chronic neck and shoulder pain, digestive issues and early signs of IBS (Irritable Bowel Syndrome). Whilst Samantha was doing everything she perceived right in terms of physical interventions (diet modifications, exercise, supplements and some medications) she had a deeper sense that her physical issues were not really stemming from her physical body. And, guess what? Samantha was correct. Issues that appear in the physical body are often actually, effectively the last port of call for a disease or illness process. Diseases do not always just start in the physical body, they start in the deeper areas of our emotions, stress levels (which are a matter of mindset and perception) and our spiritual health, which I define as how joyful we are, how connected to our life purpose, how much we live in congruence with our values. So if the illness doesn't start in the body, where does it start? Of course there is the physical aspect of a disease process due to poor nutrition and poor lifestyle and Dr Lyssa Rankin goes into great detail on this topic in her book '*Mind Over Medicine*' however for the purpose of this, we will focus on the emotions and beliefs and their link to the lack of wellbeing we experience. And the best way to do this is through examples. So back to Samantha

When Samantha came to me, I looked at all of her presenting physical symptoms and took notes, however these were not the area of focus for her sessions with me, in other words, I was not there to heal her physical issues, I was there to help with her emotional wellbeing, and the physical would take care of itself from there. I started instead, (as I do with all clients) with her emotional wellbeing, how was life for her at the stage? Did she feel happy? How did she view her overall emotional wellbeing? Let me describe the standard process I use to deal with peoples' physical issues: I start by asking what their prevailing emotions are.

---

* Name changed for privacy.

Samantha, at the time had a lot of stress in her life as she was having major issues related to living arrangements, employment, as she was miserable in her job and had a long commute to work every day. She was also continuously worried about money and constant stressed about her financial situation. When you hear of all this stress, is it any wonder she felt physically sick?

Our physical bodies are listening to the information we feed it every day and will respond to this information accordingly. Information in the form of emotions stress, nutrition etc. Once I had established the state of Samantha's emotional wellbeing, I moved on to addressing what her core limiting beliefs were? How does she perceive herself and her life?

It turns out Samantha had beliefs that were not serving or empowering her at all. Beliefs that existed were; "I am not worthy," "I am not good enough," "I am not capable," 'Bad things happen to me," "Bad things will happen in life." These beliefs had been with her throughout her entire life (created in childhood before the age of seven years of age, as is the case with all of our beliefs, both positive and negative) and these beliefs were playing out in her adult world through anxiety, stress, overwhelm, financial issues and, most predominantly, physical pain. Because, here's the thing, you cannot have good physical health if you do not have good emotional health.

So with Samantha I worked on identifying the predominant emotions and beliefs, finding when they were created and then clearing the beliefs and traumatic events and changing them for positive beliefs. The tool I work with is called Matrix Reimprinting using EFT (Emotional Freedom Technique).

Such techniques known as 'Energy Psychology' are so effective that they enable us to reduce the stress we have in our lives by adjusting our own perceptions and therefore lifting our energy to feel better and when our energy is better our bodies are better. [4]

---

[4] www.energypsych.org

This healing tool uses the process of identifying the (limiting) beliefs we have, labeling the negative emotions we feel and then using these emotions and where we feel them in our body to track where they started in our past. We are able to go back as far as being in the womb and our birth (the level of trauma we experience at birth can have a huge impact on our beliefs system and a lot of anxiety begins in the womb, carried through from mother). "Impossible!" I hear you say, not so when you understand The Mind Body connection[5] and this is when the magic starts to happen. Over a matter of sessions (six to be precise) something started to happen to Samantha's physical symptoms as we healed her emotional 'stuff', they started to reduce, and then over time, disappear. Three years on, Samantha no longer has IBS, she no longer has fibromyalgia and has incredible physical health. This is just one example of how this Mind Body healing works. But for now I want to digress and explain this further before I give more examples.

There's an aspect to physical health that needs to be touched on here. What causes us to have these limiting negative beliefs and emotions in the first place? One word, trauma. Now many people think that trauma has to be big significant life events that we remember forever, however, to a child under the age of seven a trauma can be anything. They may be seemingly insignificant to an adult but to a child things such as bullying, parents divorcing or arguing a lot, teachers picking on a child at school (a very common one I have to address in clients) the first day at school, being teased, being told off. All these mini traumas are significant to a young child. So what defines them as being traumatic? They are events that are called a U.D.I.N. And meet the following four criteria; Unexpected, Dramatic, Isolating (you feel alone and unsupportive at the time of the event) and No known resources to deal with this event at the time it occurs.

---

[5] 'The Connection' https://theconnection.tv/

When we experience these UDINs big or small, what it then does is send a shock to our system and this is when the body picks up the memory and holds a record of the event, not only in our minds as limiting perceptions and beliefs, but also in our sub conscious and in our body's cells. The research of renowned cell biologist Dr Bruce Lipton[6] has scientifically proven that our cells and their membranes carry receptors that read information from our environment and contain their own ability to hold memories.

So it is not just our mind that remembers traumatic and upsetting events, but also our body, which explains why traditional talk therapies often do not completely resolve the issues, because they are focused solely on what is going on in our minds, and ignore the physical feelings connected to these thoughts. We store this information in the outer part of our cells and this is why we can remember events from so long ago when we use the processes I describe. A popular way to explain this, is think of your favourite smells and how they can instantly remind you of happy times as a child, or what about phobias? Ask any person with a phobia to imagine the phobia, and then ask them what they feel when you mention what they are afraid of. Without even seeing the spider/snake/rat they will clearly tell you that they can actually feel the phobia in their body as cold sweats, clenched toes, heart palpitations etc. This is because the body remembers shocking events as much as the mind. The power to heal when we integrate mind and body techniques, can far surpass a reliance on physical interventions. When you consider that our bodies have billions of cells, it makes sense that working with the body can link the connection between our emotions and our physical wellbeing. It seems that scientists may have discovered the missing piece of the wellness puzzle. Sub-conscious memories connected to past events that are held in the body's memory field and then express themselves as physical symptoms and issues over time.

---

[6] The Biology of Belief by Dr Bruce Lipton

Let's use another example. Kathy had been seeing a very experienced and able naturopath nutritionist for some time to deal with her digestive issues and inability to lose weight and was wanting to do a detox program, however had doubts she would be capable of seeing it through. She was referred to me by the nutritionist, who, instinctively knew that her physical symptoms (whilst had shown some improvements) were not completely healing and that there were some underlying emotional issues inhibiting her full recovery.

Kathy came to me with a list of negative emotions and beliefs and had identified that she had anxiety and had had so for a long time (most of her life). Her anxiety always manifested as feelings in her stomach area. Along with the anxiety were combined beliefs around not being worthy, feeling not good enough, not feeling capable, being out of control, fear of not being able to do things and worried bad things would happen. Kathy had also taken on a belief that relationships were hard, and at the time she was seeing me she was having issues with her own relationship. She also wanted to return to university to do more advanced study, however she was afraid she would fail. All this worry and angst was having significant impacts on her physical wellbeing.

Together using the energy and feelings in the body that these beliefs conjured up, we worked on using this energy and what came up from her subconscious mind (which makes up 95% of all or our behaviours and habits) to track these feelings and anxiety back to her childhood and her mother. It turned out that Kathy had learned her anxiety from her mother, who herself had suffered anxiety her entire life. I cannot begin to tell you the amount of work I do for clients on the beliefs and behaviours they learn from their parents, as well as the traumas and issues that get carried from generation to generation. I cannot do this topic justice in this chapter, so I will not open that can of worms. Let it just be known, that healing often requires the acceptance that a lot of what has happened to us was written on our walls before we were born. But it is not all doom and gloom because we now have ways to address these issues. Matrix Reimprinting is just one way, but there is also family constellation work, spiritual healing and past life work that can be done.[7]

---

[7] "Many Lives Many Masters." By Dr Brian L. Weiss

Throughout the sessions, we never even addressed Kathy's actual physical illnesses and problems, we continued to work through all of her beliefs and negative emotions instead. What then began to happen, was what, in many instances people would deem a miracle. Over the next 6 sessions and in the following year Kathy's digestive issues and overall self-belief improved, to the point that she was able to complete the detox program (firstly because she believed she was capable of doing so, and secondly because her anxiety and fears had been overcome).

Subsequently, Kathy lost 15 kilos in that time! She no longer had digestive issues, but something else had begun to happen, because her relationship with herself was improving and her self-worth and self-belief had been changed to positive and empowering ones, her partner started to treat her differently. Without her ever once needing to address his behaviour, he started to respond to the difference in her energy. From this their communication improved and through her own emotional healing she was able to provide support to her partner so he could feel better about himself. Happy to say they are still together and their relationship is better than ever, and Kathy's physical health is the best it has been in years.

There is insurmountable research that supports the notion that to heal the body we must heal the mind. [8] And the absence of this understanding and way of addressing well-being also explains why seemingly healthy eaters still get illnesses. In her Book '*Mind over Medicine*' Dr Lyssa Rankin[9] studied research papers that confirmed that a happy and positive/optimistic person who drank regularly was likely to have better physical health than a stressed out anxious individual who ate well and didn't drink.

---

[8] Dr David Hamilton

[9] Dr Lyssa Rankin "Mind Over Medicine"

Why is this? Because your emotional wellbeing has a far greater impact on how healthy we will be. Add to this the new science in the study of 'Epigenetics' which means 'above genetics' and we now know that our wellbeing is so much more about our emotions, and environment and in particular our beliefs, than it is just about our genes and which ones we are born with. We are not the victims of our genetics, and the new science of 'Epigenetics' confirms this and is now informing us that there is so much more to play in illness than the genes we are born with.[10] But that is a topic for a whole different chapter. But if you are interested in this topic, check out the book "The Genie in your Genes."[11]

This realization also explains why we cannot ignore the feelings and emotions we are experiencing daily when we are trying to heal our physical issues.[12]. The work of Doctor Herbert Benson, has identified that chronic stress and the stress response is as much a cause of our physical illnesses as any poor diet or environmental triggers, and to heal our chronic stress we need to reverse it and bring about a relaxation response.

However this can be difficult to do if we do not address the underlying mindset and emotions that cause us to get stressed in the first place. Yes there could be things in our environment that are stressing us, and this can happen, but when the stress is chronic and causing us to get sick, then we have to look deeper and heal our own perceptions and emotions and past traumas so we no longer react to outside situations the way we do. Happiness literally is an inside job, as too is wellbeing.

---

[10] http://www.whatisepigenetics.com/

[11] 'The Genie in Your Genes' by Dawson Church

[12] Dr Bruce Lipton

To bring about change in our outside world we need to do the inner work first. We are getting sicker and sicker and stress is a major contributing factor to this due to the disruption it causes to our body's vital functions of repair and renewal or tissues and cells. If we have had past negative situations that have caused us stress, it is likely that similar occurring situations will cause further stressful responses, and over time instead of getting better, it just gets worse every time we are triggered. Our triggers become so engrained in our psyche that this is the only way to react to these stressful situations.

However, over time this chronic stress will be detrimental to our wellbeing. And this is why healing past events, addressing the negative perceptions through Mind Body work like EFT and Matrix Reimprinting, as well as yoga, mediation and mindfulness are so crucial to ensure our physical wellbeing has the best chance of improvement. There are no quick fixes, no pills that can cure an ill.

You in yourself have the ability to heal yourself (with the right resources) and it is not serving us to think that there is a medication out there intelligent enough to truly heal us and be responsible for our complete well-being, that is like expecting a computer to be as close to human as possible it experiences feelings and emotions like we do. It is us who have (with the right interventions and support) the ability within us to resolve the issues I have spoken of. Do you now think it profoundly uplifting and encouraging concept to know that, within you is the ability to overcome your stress, anxiety not matter what is happening outside in the world around you? It all comes down to your perception.

I always like to use the analogy of the car to compare to us as humans. When our car starts to show signs of not running well, we do not simply look at the exterior and say "Oh I think the car needs a paint job I will do that and see if that helps." We do not put on some alloy wheels and make the exterior look better hoping that this will improve the motor's performance. What we do instead is, we seek help from a professional (mechanic) and we lift the bonnet (the mind and emotions) and we get the professional to look in there and really see what is going on.

We replace the oil (negative beliefs) with new oil (positive beliefs) perhaps get the timing belt sorted (reduce stress through mindfulness and meditation) and we may even need new parts (new perceptions and habits) and then when we do this the car is likely to run better again, and so do we with a similar approach. And here's the interesting thing, have you ever noticed that even if it is pouring with rain outside or a stinking hot 40 degree day the car doesn't simply stop and say "Because of the weather today I am feeling overwhelmed, it's the rain's fault I am not working." That would never happen, the car is resilient (most often) to what is happening outside of it, and if the car does have an accident, it is often possible it will be repaired and carry on.

My father is a panel beater, and he said that more often than not, most cars can be repaired, he said some, just like people, will need a lot of work and a major overhaul, however, with the right patience, time and support, they can be rebuilt and sometimes even back to the former glory and in better condition than when they had the accident.

And that is EXACTLY how we as humans can be if we take the right steps and actions as well. Yet we as humans like to blame the outside world for our failings when really it is what is going on underneath that bonnet, that is inhibiting us from feeling complete health and well-being. But the thought of lifting that bonnet and working with alternative healers and therapists is just a little too scary and a little too overwhelming. However, fear never ever improved our quality of life.

Ever noticed how some people do not get stressed in certain situations where others will fall in a crumbling heap at the mere sight of a challenge? Why is this? Again, it comes down to your beliefs system and how we view the world. Are you an optimist or a pessimist? Do you complain a lot (because you believe and expect bad things to happen)? Or are you one to forget about it and move on, and see the positives? Whatever the situation each person's experience is subjective and unique.

Have you noticed that people who are constantly sick or in physical pain, generally do have negative outlooks on life? They are often pessimists, lack hope and tend to see the bad side of things.[13] Again why is this? Because Beliefs are the foundation of everything we do and feel. They represent how successful we will be in life, how likely we are to be well, our likelihood of having positive relationships and how we will get through life's challenges, including how likely we are to heal from illnesses and diseases[14].

Fortunately we now know that changing these beliefs will in fact mean we can completely change our current life situations. Our wellbeing improves when our outlook on life improves and we reduce our stress, and the research of Andrew Weil MD and Herbert Benson MD affirms this.

The work I do in holistic therapies using the mentioned techniques has had so many benefits for clients. There was Rebecca who had anxiety and was in a constant state of dissatisfaction over where her life was at. Because of this she experienced a lot of tension in her neck and back.

Together we worked on clearing her beliefs about not being good enough, and from there her emotions and well-being went ahead in leaps and bounds and so many of the things she wanted to manifest began to occur (like being proposed to by her fiancé).

And what about John who suffered incredible anxiety and panic attacks because he had a belief that he needed to be in control of everything, and these panic attacks meant he had to take time off work on a regular basis. We cleared these control beliefs and his panic attacks disappeared, as too did his anxiety and that only took three sessions. He did not take any medication as was suggested, there was no need.

I would just like to add here that in the case of anxiety and depression, sometimes medication is necessary to help bring some equilibrium to how we feel, however, they are not the long term solution as the previous information in this chapter explains why. Heal the emotions, heal your body.

---

[13] Mind over Medicine

[14] mindovermedicinebook.com

Lastly, a client called Denise had major self-confidence issues and was in a relationship that she did not want to be in and this was resulting in physical pain in her body, headaches and migraines. We cleared her beliefs around feeling overwhelmed and she was able to see her partner in a new light and realize her dissatisfaction was based around her own lack of self-worth. We cleared this and replaced her limiting beliefs with positive self-empowered ones and her headaches and migraines disappeared, and her relationship also improved as she was able to love her partner for who he was, because she loved herself for who she was.

One last further point I would like to make to further highlight this connection between negative beliefs and emotions and our physical issues. There is a science known as Meta Medicine, which is a diagnostic tool that tells us that each physical issue/pain/disease/illness has a very specific set of underlying trauma/s and belief/s systems. As well as explaining what emotions and beliefs we need to be looking for to heal specific issues in the body.[15]

This scientific tool is also affirmed in the spiritual world by Medical intuitives and mediums (people who can tell a person what has caused their physical problem through reading their energy field) such as world renowned Caroline Myss and Anthony Williams.

These people are also able to identify the same disease causes as the science of META Medicine does.[16] A brilliant book by Inna Segal[17] also explains the Mind body connection, and the most obvious and simplified one we know of is *'You Can Heal Your Life'* by Louise Hay. I have mentioned other resources at the bottom of this chapter.[18] There are typical places in the body where we feel specific emotional issues, a few common ones are:

- Anxiety - felt in the stomach, digestive issues
- Heart break or sadness –the heart or chest area,

---

[15] www.metamedicine.se/what-is-meta-medicine/

[16] "Anatomy of the Spirit" by Caroline Myss, "Medical Medium" by Anthony William

[17] The Secret Language of the Body by Inna Segal

[18] Why am I sick? By Richard Flook and 'The Biogenealogy Sourcebook" by Christian Fleche

- Fear of death or unresolved sadness through grief and loss - the lungs,
- Carrying burdens (supporting others to point of feeling stressed) – the shoulders,
- Fear of lack of support (emotional of financial) - the lower back,
- Issues with moving forward in life or what direction to take - present in the lower limbs, knees, feet etc (which is why so many elderly have hip issues once they retire).

So whilst none of this Mind Body healing is new, it is now becoming so much more accessible and acceptable. It is my absolute understanding and belief through studying the literature and working with clients, that it is the missing piece of the healing puzzle. Until we begin to see the whole healing journey as 'holistic' too many of us will continue to die of cancers and other diseases. Whilst there is no guarantee that doing this 'inner work' will help you overcome your disease, it certainly cannot make you any sicker and it most certainly will ensure that your emotional wellbeing does improve, and surely that can only be a good thing?

The mindset we need to get our head around is, healing takes commitment, it requires a willingness to go beyond conventional, it takes trust and optimism and a willingness to step outside the common approaches, and an investment in ourselves. If popping a pill cured us, we would not die of these diseases we get treated for. Alternative therapies are giving so much more hope to so many, and improving the quality of lives in the thousands. It is now a case of talking about this openly, and educating people on the possibilities. It is not about putting down one treatment or the other it is about integration, working together, eastern with western, emotional with physical. If we can be open to this approach, so many more of us will live to see ripe old ages, or at least die knowing we feel better having tried everything available to us. I have hope, and that in itself can heal.

By Sonja Courtis

About the author

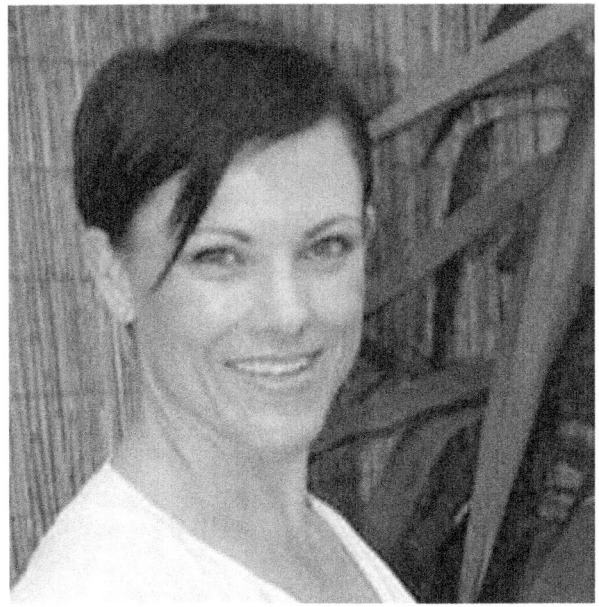

My name is Sonja Courtis, born in New Zealand.
I am a specialist in assisting people overcome stress, anxiety and depression. I help people identify the underlying causes of their current emotional issues and treat underlying traumas that have lead to current states of anxiety and depression.
I am trained in:
NLP - Neuro Linguistic Programming.
EFT – Emotional Freedom Technique
And Matrix Reimprinting (using EFT)
I have 24 years experience in the field of studying psychology, spirituality, META health research as well as a qualified secondary teacher specializing in working with children with trauma backgrounds, special needs and behavioural issues.

I embarked on the journey of helping others after the death of my brother to suicide when he was 15 years old (I was 17) and that has taken be on a personal immersion into the field of understanding human psychological and physical illness and in particular issues of mental health. This lead me to train in the Energy Psychology field as I believe these new sciences are the missing piece to helping more people overcome anxiety and depression.

I have assisted 100s of people in seeking help with their stress and anxiety disorders.

www.healthyandhealed.co.nz
www.facebook.com/healthyandhealed
instagram - healthyhealed

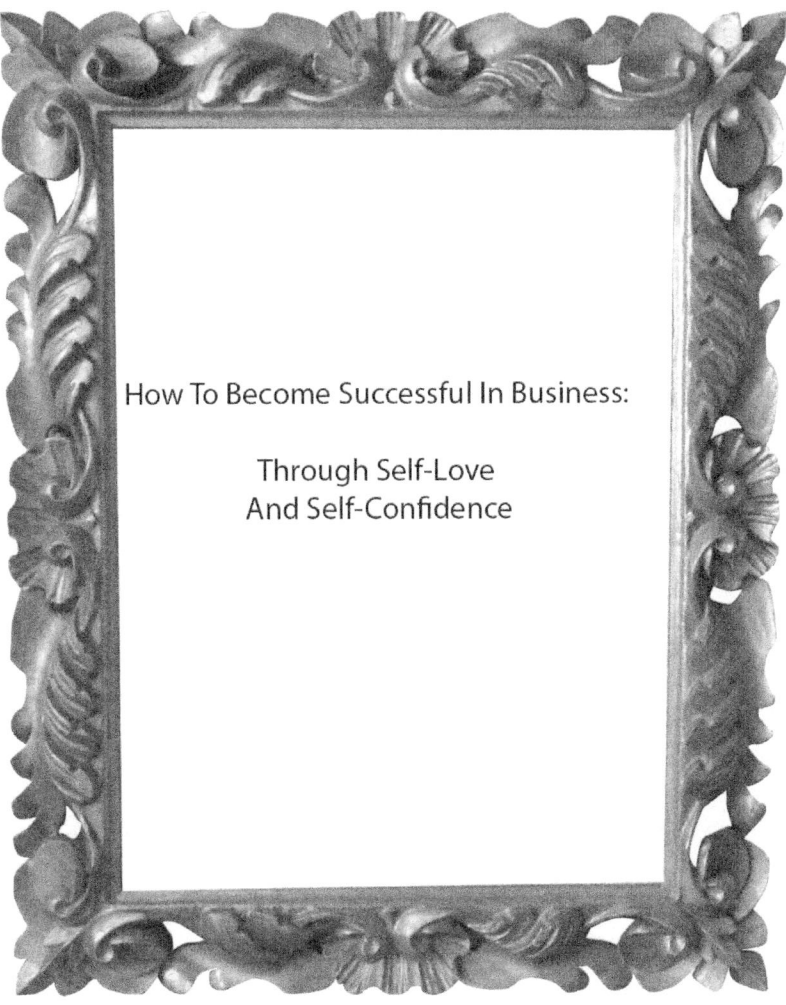

How To Become Successful In Business:

Through Self-Love
And Self-Confidence

How To Become Successful In Business: Through Self-Love And Self-Confidence

We all strive to want the best that life has to offer. It is this natural human instinct in all of us that drives us to want to be successful in both business and in our personal life. In order to achieve this ~~success~~, you will need to learn how.

The first thing you should know about success is that it is something you must do for yourself. It requires hard graft, commitment and determination.

If you have the courage to look within yourself and truly understand who you are and what you are capable of, then you are already on the right path. Being honest about yourself is the first step. In this chapter I will be discussing how self-love and self-confidence can help you to be successful in business.

Now, let us get to the important stuff!

SELF-LOVE

Self-love is essential for your mental and physical health and the health of your business.

Self-love is about fully and unconditionally accepting yourself for who you are and what you have become so far. Self-love can assist those less confident with removing the suffocating mask you wear for the rest of the world. It reflects a deep realisation that you are enough.

Everything in your reality is your own projection and nothing can stop you from effortlessly fulfilling your dreams.

Despite the fact that self-love can help you heal, grow and succeed, some harmful myths prevent entrepreneurs from practising it. Here are some of the most common myths:

- **Self-love will make me selfish**

On some level, you understand that self-love is beneficial. So why don't you try it?

Caring for oneself is frequently confused with being narcissistic or self-centred, many people are hesitant to practise self-love. If you neglect yourself, you could find yourself experiencing a lack of focus, low energy, low motivation and irritability. This in turn will lead to all aspects of your life being turned upside down.

Self-love assists you in setting appropriate boundaries, allowing you to feel positive and confident. When you prioritise taking time for yourself, you feel better about yourself and your business benefits from it.

- **Self-love will hinder my progress**

Another common misconception about self-love is that if you slow down and take the time to heal yourself, you will become lazy and unimaginative. We know it is beneficial to take a step back and embrace stillness in order to know your true self. This does not necessarily mean that your progress will cease. In fact it will improve and prosper.

In reality you will become more creative, spontaneous, intuitive and inspired. When you are in fight-or-flight mode, your memory, emotional expression, judgment, impulse control, problem solving, social interaction and motor functioning are all impaired serving no purpose. When you reveal your true self, free of anxiety, doubts and insecurities, you do a far better job because you are no longer in this negative mode.

Many business owners are afraid of slowing down and missing opportunities. But the truth is that there are many things in this world over which you have no control and it is sometimes beneficial to take a deep breath and place trust in yourself.

- **Self-love will render me weak**

Society often sees life in black and white. There is the misconception that self-love equals weakness. If you believe this, then now is time to change and update your mind set. Self-love when practised can propel you to new heights of success.

Self-love entails accepting your limitations unconditionally and not being ashamed of them. Being able to accept yourself completely without judgment is probably the most difficult thing you will ever practise. When I see someone shouting or acting aggressively, I think of them as weak and fragile. I view them as bullies who threaten and intimidate others in order to feel strong and superior. In the corporate world we have become accustomed to bullying being a sign of strength. Correspondingly, acts of kindness are misinterpreted as signs of weakness.

However, when you are kind to yourself, you can better regulate your emotions. Accepting all aspects of yourself, good and bad, is the ultimate freedom and leadership style you should prioritise in personal and professional relationships. I know many people are prone to criticising their own limitations and flaws but from my experience they should instead strive for unconditional acceptance. Self-love will not make you weak. Rather, it will strengthen and improve your confidence and ability immeasurably.

So, make a list of things you keep hidden from others or are embarrassed about. Then, to avoid feeling overwhelmed, start accepting one limitation at a time by telling yourself, "I love you despite this limitation" as often as you can. This will assist you in becoming whole. At the end of the day, we all want to be unconditionally accepted and you can do that for yourself.

How Self-Love Can Aid Business Success

Running a business is already stressful, with the constant marketing, holding onto and increasing your client database and keep creating fresh content. Keeping abreast of the ever-changing social media platforms can be overwhelming and time consuming. Add further responsibilities such as a partner, children and family to the mix and you have entered the feast or famine cycle.
I'm not trying to be negative. Not at all!
I want you to take a deep breath, stop whatever else it is you are juggling. Put the kettle on! Relax and read on.
I am not just talking about sumptuous bubble baths and early nights (although I do highly recommend them). I'm referring to developing a strong relationship with yourself.
Unless you are generating a comfortable automated passive income, your business needs you and investing time in yourself is one of the best ways to ensure you and your business stay consistently healthy and on top form. Understandably, you are probably wondering where you are going to schedule time for yourself in an already hectic day. Bear with me.
Self-Love means you:

- **Regularly prioritise yourself and your business!**

Even the airlines tell us that we must first put on *our* own oxygen masks. Putting ourselves first becomes easier when we practise self-love. You will realise that prioritising your own needs over those of your partner, children and parents etc. benefits everyone equally in the long run.

Okay, I'm not saying you put yourself first "all the time" or neglect your children. I just mean that you make it clear that you and your business have requirements. After all, the success of your business could be the family's ticket to financial independence. You will, for example, be able to send your children to the best schools, take amazing holidays, even allow your partner to retire early. This does not happen overnight and it certainly will not happen if you frequently drop everything to attend to their every need.

Do what needs to be done to lessen your guilt for feeling not to be always there for everyone. Hire a cleaning service, employ a babysitter/carer, ask for help, delegate.

Keep your partner, family, business associates informed of your big vision and that you will not always be available. Make a space where you can work with the least amount of distraction.

Also, don't forget! Self-care for you and your business means taking time to unwind.

- **Give yourself permission to dream big**

When you practise self-love, you are simultaneously strengthening your self-belief and confidence muscles. They work together and act as a team. Self-love allows you not only to know that your business dreams are achievable but also to take action to make them a reality.

- **Establish clear boundaries and speak up**

Following on from the previous two points, ensure that when you say yes, you are not saying no to yourself.

The more *no's*, the less time and space you will have for your *yeses* and dream clients. Do not feel obligated to take on additional work or clients who are less than ideal.

Continue to practise saying what you mean. Allow your yes to be yes and your no to be no. Ask yourself whether it is in line with your ideal lifestyle and business vision.

- **Make more sound business decisions**

The more we practise self-love the more we are drawn to activities that provide us with clarity. The more practise, the more creative you will become. Amazing ideas will flow and develop and in turn generate further income.
We are less likely to do something simply because others in our industry are doing it. When we listen to our gut instinct, we have a strong relationship with ourselves. We become more genuine and allow ourselves to be guided by what we truly believe in.

- **Make a name for yourself in your industry**

The more you practise self-love, the more you accept and embrace your quirks and what distinguishes you from the competition. You will highlight what distinguishes you from everyone else and makes you stand out.
You will create a brand that truly represents YOU. It sounds simple but allowing yourself to be true to your business and to choose your own style from the clothes, fonts, website and images that reflect YOU is a game-changer. Your ideal clients will see you as a beacon.

- **Recognise that you are not for everyone**

There will always be the possibility of negativity from someone either trolling online with nothing better to do or a self-proclaimed friend who will comment unfavourably on you and your business.
The more you love yourself, the less this will affect you. You will develop a thicker skin and any comments will be water off a duck's back.
As a result, putting yourself out there on social media will feel less intimidating. Your business perspective is not going to be everyone's "cup of tea", some people will not understand your vision. This is not your problem.

- **Prioritise your health and life balance**

Self-love implies that you will not work every waking hour. It means you will be gentler with yourself. You are not a robot. If you do not get enough sleep or nutrition and very little exercise and fresh air (not to mention fun) your business and you will suffer.
The more you practise self-love the better you will take care of yourself because it will become a habit.
Remember that self-love motivates you to do more of what you enjoy. This includes spending quality time with your loved ones.
Now you can see why I said it was a win-win situation for your children, partner, family and friends.
So, the next time you find yourself burning the candle at both ends, take a moment to reflect on what YOU want and need and then give it to yourself guilt-free.

SELF-CONFIDENCE

Have you ever felt like an imposter? I have.
You are up to your ears with responsibilities, doing everything you can to meet your objectives and manage your stress, when that nagging (but familiar) thought hits you: Who are you trying to fool?
Perhaps you lack the necessary skills to pursue your dreams. Those feelings of inadequacy and uncertainty are terrifying. However, they are most likely based on preconceived thoughts.
You are probably underestimating your ability to achieve your goals and pursue your dreams in life. This can cause a lot of fear and anxiety and in the worst-case scenario, paralysis.
If only you could learn to be more self-confident, like the people you admire. You certainly can! Continue reading to find out how.

Self-Confidence Is Priceless but Many of Us Struggle to Achieve it

Work ethic, ambition and dedication will get you far but confidence can mean the difference between a mediocre result and a massively successful one.
Your financial success is heavily influenced by how much you believe in your own abilities and how well you present that belief to others.
Being confident inspires confidence in others, which is important when looking for a new business partner or new clients because you can't expect others to believe in you if you don't believe in yourself.
Therefore, assertiveness is widely regarded as a desirable trait. It has an impact on almost every aspect of your life, which raises some difficult questions:

- Why do so many of us have difficulty with this?
- More importantly, what can we do to make it better?

Most Confidence Advice Is Confusing and Unhelpful

"You should be more self-assured!"
You have probably heard that advice more times than you can count. When I hear someone say this it always makes me cringe. I want to face them and ask the obvious question: *How?*
We are all aware of the importance of confidence. The problem is understanding how to achieve it. Some people believe it is "acquired" from birth. Confident people are often unable to explain how they obtained this advantageous trait articulately.
The good news is that confidence can be learnt. You, like me, can consciously develop it to help achieve what you want in life.

Practical Ways to Begin Increasing Your Confidence

This is not a quick fix or a process that can be completed overnight. It may take some time to shake off the uncertainty and old habits and reveal the stronger, more confident *"you"*.

But the effort is well worth it.

Here's how to begin:

- **Be the best version of yourself**

I wasted years trying to work out how to fix my confidence issues from within.
If I had approached the problem differently and decided to start from the outside, I could have saved myself grief, time and toil!
You may not be able to change your feelings about yourself overnight but you can change how you are perceived from the outside. You could consider focusing more on your personal image and appearance. If you feel good about how you look this inevitably will boost your self-confidence.
You do not have to spend a fortune on an expensive wardrobe or extravagant treatments. How do you dress when you are at your most confident? It does not have to be formal but it should be clean and respectable, in keeping with the business you wish to portray. Make every effort to convey your own vision of success through how you look.
People will respond positively if you appear self-assured and positive, giving you more reason to feel and act confidently.

- **Be aware of your speech, posture and body language**

Think about the most confident person you know. For me, it is my Mum. Now answer the following:
- Do they slouch?
- Do they speak rapidly afraid of being cut off?
- Is their working environment shambolic?

People who are confident do not behave in this manner. Their posture is excellent and would make any mother proud! They communicate with open, confident body language. They typically speak slowly and clearly, so that you do not need to ask them to repeat themselves.

There is no reason why you can't improve on these points regardless of how you feel about yourself. You have complete control over them and it will give you a boost of confidence.

Take note of your:
- **Speech:** Experiment with speaking slowly and loudly enough to be heard. There are numerous exercises you can try to improve your performance. One of my favourites is to record myself recounting a familiar story, taking care not to rush and leaving room for natural pauses. You could even join a public speaking club.
- **Posture:** Stand up straight, head high and shoulders back! According to a study paper published in 2010 in the journal Psychological Science by Dana Carney and Andy Yap from Columbia University and Amy Cuddy from Harvard University, *"upright, expansive posture makes people feel and act more powerful than guarded, closed posture"*.
- **Nonverbal communication:** Pay close attention to how you interact with others. Avoid fidgeting or looking around instead make direct eye contact with your peers.

This may feel strange at first but persevere. With practice you will become more at ease and it will start to feel much more natural.

- **Surround yourself with positive and supportive environment**

Your surroundings have a greater impact on your attitude to work and life than you may realise. It can either encourage your confidence to grow or erode it day after day.

This means you can give yourself the gift of more confidence simply by being particular about who and what you surround yourself with.

Examine the people and the environment in which you spend the most time. Are you surrounded by positive, optimistic people who strive to improve themselves and achieve their goals? Or are they quick to dismiss and disparage any innovative ideas or successful people? Is the atmosphere conducive to a productive outcome? Do you find inspiration from your surroundings?

The media you consume is also important. Stop reading clickbait gossip stories or negative news stories about political candidates you despise!

Remove negative people and messages in your life and replace them with positive people and content that inspires you (podcasts, books, etc.).

- **Exercise**

In addition to physical and mental benefits, physical activity can boost your confidence.

Exercise causes a flood of endorphins in your body, which can improve your self-image and alleviate stress. It does not require two-hour workouts. A little bit will get you a long way.

If you continue to exercise and live a healthy lifestyle, you will begin to notice the physical changes which will bolster your confidence.

- **Clearly visualise your desired outcomes**

Visualisation is extremely powerful but most of us abuse it. We let our anxious minds run wild with disaster scenarios leaving no room for success. Experts believe that visualising the desired outcome ahead of time will boost your confidence because it prepares your brain for success.
Why not give it a try?
Visualise your success for the next significant event in your business. The clearer and more detailed your vision, the better. What are you wearing? What are your thoughts? Is there anyone else in the room?
Imagine your goals as if you have already accomplished them and your confidence will skyrocket.

- **Look for small victories**

Many people struggle with confidence because they are too focused on the end result. That massive success you so desperately desire may appear far removed from reality but it is attainable.
To achieve success you will need a great deal of optimism, positivity and self-assurance which is all achievable by building on it gradually.
Divide your goals into small, manageable chunks, preferably with outcomes under your control and focus on what you need to do today.
One of my biggest mistakes when I first started my business was attempting to earn a specific amount of money per month. You may have similar benchmark in mind. The issue I had was that the amount seemed so far away. It was difficult to make £100, let alone thousands, when I was still learning to work things out.
Things became much easier after I reduced my goals, organising and prioritising those targets which would help me in the now and benefit my future long term. I concentrated on what I needed to do at the time rather than focus solely on the future outcome.
Your daily victories will add up to weekly and monthly triumphs. As your results improve you will create a pattern of success and with this your confidence will go from strength to strength.

- **Make gratitude a daily habit**

You may desire so much more from your business and life but what about all the possessions you have accumulated over the years as your business goes from strength to strength?

It is all too easy to get caught up in the single minded and overzealous attitude for immediate success. This can come at a cost. Without acknowledging all your strengths which got you to where you are and which have kept you on an even keel, you risk the possibility of losing what is most important to you.

There is no reason why you cannot appreciate what you have already accomplished, how far you have come and the people who have supported you along the way.

Practicing gratitude is extremely simple. It could be as simple as listing five things you are grateful for after you wake up or just before you go to bed.

What you are grateful for each day will change but your past accomplishments will continue to be a reminder how far you have come and sustain your confidence.

Some people maintain a gratitude journal. But I prefer to reflect on what I'm thankful for before I go to bed. There is no "correct" way to do this other than a routine that works best for you. Make expressing gratitude a habit and you will feel less anxious and more confident.

When you are grateful it is impossible to feel afraid. Try it out and see for yourself!

There is no better time than now to begin building your confidence. It takes time, but the process builds on itself. Small and consistent gains result in better decisions and opportunities, success and an increase in confidence. It turns into a self-sustaining cycle which will help you overcome anxiety and worry, pursue your dreams relentlessly and overcome obstacles that will inevitably arise along the way.

Amber Asghar

About the author

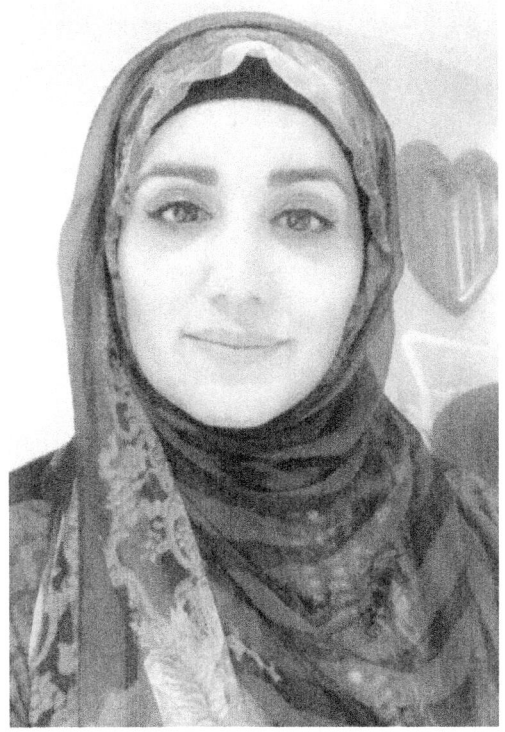

Multi-talented Amber Asghar is a self-made career woman and a mother of four children.
Ambitious from an early age, she left school at the age of sixteen in order to devote her time to build a business career.

The business woman

After joining the family luxury fashion store, Amber was ready to open her own fashion and fabric business by her twenties. She specialised in soft furnishings and turned her hand to interior design, decorating hotels and homes.
She also had a stint in the jewellery business, starting her own gold and diamond business within her family's 24 ct gold jewellery shop, designing exquisite bespoke pieces.

Amber's real love has been in property however, ever since she set eyes on her dream house at the age of fifteen.
She vowed to own such a luxury home by the time she reached her thirties - realising her dream at the age of 32.
The achievement spurred her on to invest in real estate, and she now owns and manages several properties.

The Crypto specialist

Amber belongs to the mere 3.9 % women who are at present engaged in the crypto business. Women only made up 1% of the industry when she started. She is a passionate and successful crypto currency investor who has helped many others with her advice.

Holistic Skin & Wellness Therapist

Amber isn't only an astute and successful businesswoman. She has a strong spiritual side and credits her achievements in business to visualisation techniques that she has been practising since the age of twelve.
Her belief in treating the body, mind and soul to achieve all around health led to an interest in holistic wellness therapies and in particular the skin. Skin is the first organ to show signs of distress and unhappiness. Amber's experience with skincare comes from her own personal journey where stress and a hectic lifestyle played a part in a number of skin issues.
Her passion for skincare led Amber to qualify as a professional facial therapist. She works only with skincare products that are based on natural ingredients and do not contain any harmful chemicals. She offers individual bespoke facials in her exclusive treatment rooms in Luton, Bedfordshire, and also undertakes private visits to give facials in the comfort of her clients' homes.

Author

The loss of a mother, who was Amber's inspiration throughout her life, was the catalyst for her recently published book Healing & Acceptance – The Path to Self-Love and Improvement.

The book explores the healing process whether the hurt was caused by childhood trauma, broken relationship or the grief from losing one's closest. It also offers invaluable advice on how to grow one's self-confidence to achieve success and a fulfilling life.

The book is available on Amazon
https://www.amazon.co.uk/Healing-Acceptance-Path-Self-Love-Improvement/dp/6277505599/ref=asc_df_6277505599/

Amber is now working on more book projects. She has a book on Crypto investment in the pipeline, as well as one on the science and treatment of skin.

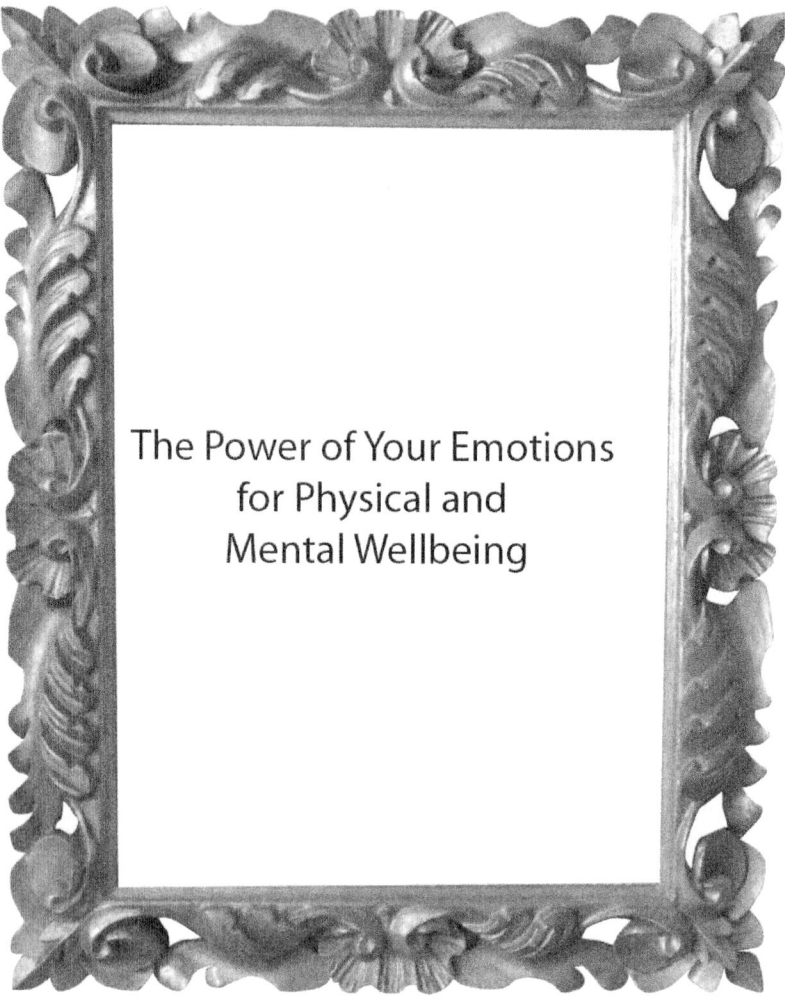

The Power of Your Emotions for Physical and Mental Wellbeing

The Power of Your Emotions for Physical and Mental Wellbeing

Your emotions have the ability to lift you up, energise you and improve your physical and mental wellbeing, therefore listening and staying in tune with what your emotions are telling you is vital to your health and state of mind.

We all harness the ability to support our mental and physical wellbeing by being in touch with our body and processing our emotions, but rarely are we taught how. In Western society there is a huge focus on doing, and very little emphasis put on simply being and truly understanding the body as a whole.

The mind is the ruler and given the upmost importance when it comes to learning and succeeding in life. Society teaches us to be focused on what you think and pays little attention to how you feel in any given moment. Our thoughts dictate our choices and living with a head driven focus has contributed to a real disconnect between what the body is trying to communicate to us.

Therefore, we get stuck in a cycle of doing, constantly striving and pushing ourselves forward, placing external needs of achievement or other people's feelings above our own. That's why the majority of people when asked the question 'What do you need right now' simply don't know how to answer.

Our emotions are there as the body's way to communicate with us, just as the mind has thoughts, the body has feelings. They can be there as a warning signal to what is going on around us, as well as letting us know what we like and dislike.

Extreme situations such as a life threatening scenario or even a really scary film, make it easy for us to understand what emotion is coming through. The problem arises in our day to day living, we either don't know how to interpret those signals from the body or we don't want to.

Emotions are often categorized as either 'good' or 'bad'. The good emotions like joy, happiness, love, peace, calm are those everyone wishes to welcome in. The 'bad' emotions such as anger, sadness, frustration, fear are ones we tend to want to ignore and shut off.

I explain to my clients that emotions are neutral, neither good or bad but simply a message from the body to be recognised and processed, and it is in fact our judgements around emotions that creates the problem. For example, someone may have been told growing up that anger was not an acceptable emotion to show, and so they find it hard to read that message from their body. Likewise, society can give us rules around how and when to show emotions. Often men don't like to get upset as it is seen as 'weak' and we all know the saying 'big boys don't cry'. This in turn means they are unable to embrace their feelings of sadness.

The problem comes because, as Brene Brown, American Research Professor and Author, says 'You cannot selectively numb your emotions'.

When we ignore the emotions we decide aren't comfortable, we also keep ourselves from fully feeling the emotions that make us feel good and we would like to have in our lives.

There are three common ways we try and avoid emotions we deem as unsuitable or uncomfortable.

1. Distraction - whether it be watching TV, scrolling on social media or playing video games, we use external stimulus to mean we don't have to face what is coming up for us.
2. Numbing out - either through food, alcohol or drugs is another way we can tune out from sitting with and processing our emotions. This technique gives us short term relief from facing what emotions are going on underneath the surface.
3. Thinking rather than feeling - you find it really easy to talk about a situation or event but what happens is you get caught in circles going over and over it because you are avoiding dropping into your

body and actually noticing what emotions are there that need to be processed and healed.

Because the body believes our emotions are important messages the problem with ignoring them is that they don't go away. Instead, they either get louder and more intense to really try and get our attention, or they can show up in the form of physical symptoms. Think headaches, back pain, nausea, whilst all of these can have a physical root cause, they can also sometimes be linked to an underlying emotional connection.

Even tense shoulders can release once the feelings of stress or overwhelm are acknowledged.

As well as getting more intense or showing up in the form of physical ailments, emotions that are ignored become trapped - causing disruption to the body's natural energy system.

You only have to think of children as a perfect example of how emotions should work. Small children can go through a variety of emotions in a very short period of time, think screaming one minute and smiling happily the next. Why? Because they are allowing their emotions to pass through without judgement and without shoving them down and ignoring them. Emotions are designed to be fluid, to show up and share their message and to release once they have been acknowledged and heard.

At the end of the day a messenger doesn't have to keep knocking at the door once the letter has been delivered. It is the same with emotions.

As adults, we don't find it as easy to honour the emotions that present to us, plus we have spent so many years becoming detached from our body we rarely reconise them. This results in emotions building up, shifting into physical symptoms as mentioned above, or simply disrupting the body's natural energy flow. Have you ever noticed when you have a big cry you suddenly feel so much lighter? That's no coincidence, it's because you've released a heavy load of emotions that you were holding on to.

Picture it like putting down a big heavy backpack that you didn't even realise you were carrying around with you, instant relief.

Signs that you are carrying unprocessed emotions around can look like:

Disproportionate reactions to situations - your emotional bank is full so it's easy to boil over and explode

Malaise and exhaustion from carrying around the emotions so your body feels heavy

Lack of motivation, wanting to withdraw from life and lacking in creative spark

None of these are conducive to supporting optimal physical and mental wellbeing. The good news is this doesn't have to be your reality and it's possible to learn to be in harmony with your body and the emotions it is giving you on a daily basis.

So where can you start?

A first step is about creating the space within your day to check in with yourself and your body to notice what emotions and sensations are showing up for you. This helps you to start coming down from your mind and once again connecting with your whole being. In these moments, getting used to asking yourself what you need, whether that be a glass of water, some food or a hug, means you are beginning to understand and respond to the signals from your body.

When we can meet our needs on a regular basis we can increase our happiness and overall wellbeing because we are listening to what feels good for us in that moment, as opposed to being guided by what we think we have to or should do.

This also allows us to start tuning in to our likes and dislikes, and the more we can recognise how we respond to different activities, jobs, or even people, the more we can begin to filter out the things that don't make us feel good. This in turn enriches our mental health because we are doing things that make us feel happy and thus energised, meaning it has a positive effect on our physical state also.

We then need to really focus on being able to name and recognise the different emotions we are feeling throughout our days and weeks. When we know how we feel this in turn strengthens our ability to give ourselves what we need.

Again, if we think of emotions as a message, once that message is acknowledge then emotions can pass through. Therefore, the more we recognise our individual feelings, the more we are able to process what doesn't feel good to open us up to more happiness, joy and gratitude.

I focus on the three A rule for allowing your emotions to guide and support. Acknowledge, Accept and Appreciate.

Acknowledging an emotion is your first step to allowing yourself to be set free from it. This can look like naming the type of emotion you are feeling, for example 'I am sad', to also recognising any physical sensations in your body, such as a tightness in your chest.

Sometimes simply honouring and acknowledging the emotion that is showing up for you can be enough to help it reduce and release. If it is still there then the next step is to allow acceptance for it.

The urge is often to want to ignore or push away uncomfortable feelings, how many times have you felt anxious but rather than leaning in to it you've attempted to get rid of it?

This can work as a temporary fix at times but what we resist persists so if we want true physical and mental wellbeing being able to allow emotions to be there rather than trying to fight them lessens the hold the emotion has on you. Close your eyes, notice where the feeling is in your body and breathe into it, giving it space to be rather than closing it off.

Thirdly, it's all about appreciating the emotion for wanting to communicate with you. We all know the saying 'don't shoot the messenger', so don't be cross with how you're feeling. Thank the emotion because without it you wouldn't know someone had treated you badly or that a situation mattered to you.

When we ignore how we feel it can lead to us allowing ourselves to be mistreated by someone, staying in situations that don't make us happy, or putting up with things because we don't know what else we would want instead. It's impossible to be mentally and physically thriving when in these situations, so the recognition that something isn't right is a powerful way to take back control not only of your life but of your physical and mental wellbeing.

Whilst we can often think that feeling into uncomfortable emotions will bring us down and keep us stuck it is quite the opposite. Feeling sadness, worry or fear, allowing it to be there and to move through you, actually allows you to then get to a place of feeling happy, relaxed and safe far more quickly.

Too often we think we can force ourselves to the feel-good states of being, and whilst on the surface it may appear that's the case, underneath there is a void because it is a forced sense of being happy rather than a true essence of it.

We must remember emotions are not to be feared, they are actually our friend and if we can allow ourselves to connect in with them regularly, we can save ourselves from more serious mental health experiences.

Anxiety and depression are often caused by a disconnect within ourselves and a build up of not honouring how we are feeling or being too afraid to deal with our emotions over a period of time.

Think of it like a boiling pot on the stove, if you turn the temperature down regularly or let the steam out it keeps bubbling away nicely, but if you ignore it and the temperature and steam builds up then the pot will eventually boil over.

The same goes for you and your emotions.

Duality exists in the whole of life, just like you can't have night without day or hot without cold, you can't experience true happiness without sadness, love without hurt and safety without fear. The beauty of this is by allowing in the 'darkness', the emotions that feel uncomfortable, it opens us up to be able to embrace even more fully the pure joy and happiness when it is here.

To live a fulfilling and wholesome life, it's vital we embrace all parts of ourselves. That is the ingredient to real lasting mental and physical wellbeing.

By Samantha Quemby

About the author

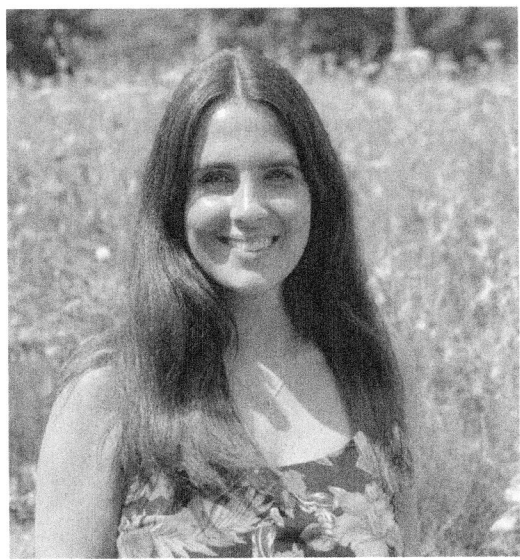

Samantha is a Performance & Life Coach who supports female entrepreneurs to banish their mindset blocks and work through past traumas to hit their goals and build the life and business they desire.

She is trained in Neurolinguistic Programming (NLP), Emotional Freedom Technique (EFT), Hypnosis, Life Coaching and Matrix Reimprinting and uses a mixture of these modalities within my coaching.

Samantha is passionate about supporting the women I work with to cultivate the feeling of success from the inside and to break free from the constant search for external validation.

Her mission is to empower women to build a business that feels good for them, creates the fulfillment and freedom they crave, and leaves burnout behind! Prior to starting her own business, Samantha Quemby Coaching, she worked as a Psychology Practitioner for The Optimum Health Clinic where she supported clients with Chronic Fatigue Syndrome with their healing journey.

Within her 7 years of coaching she has supported over 100 clients.

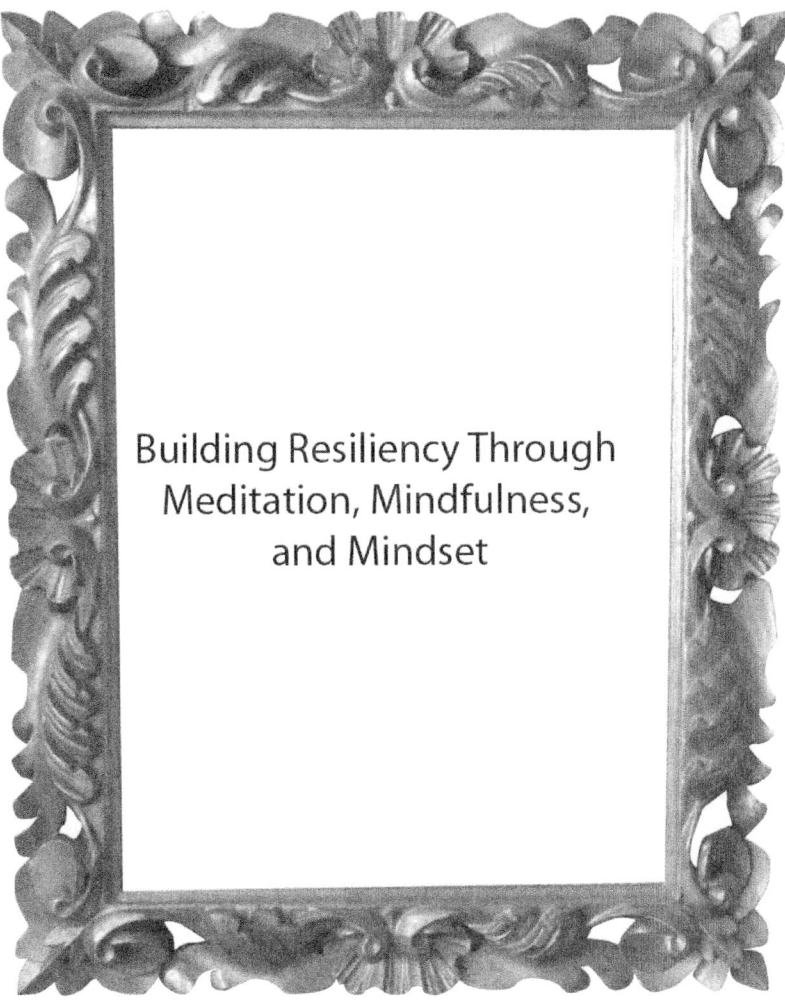

Building Resiliency Through Meditation, Mindfulness, and Mindset

Building Resiliency Through Meditation, Mindfulness, and Mindset

Resilience is like a muscle that can be refined and enhanced. The tools and methods you can use to build that resilience muscle is mediation, mindfulness and mindset. The three work together, building upon one another.

Meditation

Meditation is the practice of quieting your mind and being mindful. Meditation was a game-changer for me. It helps clear my mind, which in turn helps me deal with stress much more effectively. It can be hard to get started and I know many people feel like they're not doing it right. I felt the same way. You can start by meditating for just 3-5 minutes each day and then gradually keep increasing your time. I'm now at 11-15 minutes and I want more!! I look forward to meditation as much as I look forward to my physical workouts – strong mind, strong body. Several apps can help you get started, including Insight Timer (what I currently use), Head Space (what I used to use), and Calm. Many people claim that meditation doesn't work for them. They can't do it; they don't know how or they can't find the time. I was the same way. Here are some tips on how you can get started and incorporate a daily meditation practice into your life.

1. Start small with 1-3 minutes of meditation.
2. Use an app and select a short, guided meditation.
3. If you prefer meditating without an app, set a timer for 1-3 minutes and sit in silence and focus on your breathing. Breathe in for a count of 4, hold for 4 counts and breathe out for 4. Repeat this process 10 times.
4. Don't overthink the process. It literally means to think about nothing and clear your mind. When you do have thoughts, just realize it and let it go.
5. Establish a daily routine, either right before bed or right after your workout. Select a time that you know you can stick to and try to do it for 3-5 days in a row to get started.
6. Once you establish the habit, notice how you deal with stress and how you react to certain events.

For me, meditation has completely changed the way I react to stressful events. I find that I am much more grounded and even-keeled.

Gratitude

Cultivate a gratitude practice. I have found that having a daily practice of identifying those areas of your life where you are truly grateful can have a profound effect on your attitude and mindset. From your home and family to something as simple as a beautiful flower you saw on a walk can be part of your gratitude list. This type of practice can also help you to be more mindful and present. You will look for things to appreciate and express gratitude for, such as someone who held the door open for you or finding a heart-shaped stone. My own gratitude practice involves journaling for two minutes each day. Here's what it includes:

- Three things I'm grateful for

- Three things that went well yesterday
- Three things I could improve
- Three top goals for the day

Why these areas? It has helped me to celebrate my successes but also note where I can improve and do better. For example, sometimes I am overly anxious or in a rush for no reason. Self-awareness and personal development are critical components of mindset as well.

Understand Your 'Why'

When it comes to self-care and losing weight, your overall goals need to go beyond aesthetics. It's not enough to fit into your favorite jeans or look good for a class reunion or wedding. Looking great in a bikini is wonderful, but dig deeper. *Why* do you want to lose weight?

If you're a career-driven professional, you can't rise to the top of your profession and also serve your family well without taking care of yourself. Beyond your dream body, think about your health, your energy level and your ability to take care of yourself and others.

If you're drinking five cups of coffee a day, hitting the vending machine for your meals and drinking your calories at happy hour, that is not a sustainable, healthy lifestyle. Those habits will not allow you to be your best or to function at your best. You deserve only the best, and when you begin to honor yourself and treat your body with respect, everyone around you will follow suit.

When you think about your diet and eating habits, think about fueling your body with only the best. If you had an expensive Maserati or Lamborghini, you would fuel it with premium gasoline. Well, your body is no different. It deserves only the best so it can perform at its best.

Motivation & Goals

Everyone has different goals. It could be to lose weight, to run a 5k, to exercise without back pain or to have the energy to play with your kids or your grandkids. Figuring out your "why" is critical when it comes to motivation and achieving your goals. For every goal you choose for yourself, ask "why" until you get to the true root of your goal's purpose. This will help you stay motivated and focused. Here are some examples to help you:

Goal	Why
I want to lose weight.	It will help me feel better in clothes, have more energy, increase my confidence, and reduce my cholesterol and blood pressure. I want to be healthier as I get older so I can keep up with my kids and to be a good role model.
I want to run a 5k.	I've never run more than a block and I want to see if mentally/physically, I can achieve this goal. It will help me stick with my workout plan. My spouse is a runner and it could help us become closer.

Aesthetics are nice and are an added bonus as you strive to get healthier, but they cannot dictate your goals. In addition, a number on the scale—while a great measurement and progress tool—is also not a great motivator. Instead, ask yourself: what will losing 20 or 50 pounds do for you? I would imagine you would have more confidence. You would feel good about your body and you look good in clothes. You would have more energy. From a health perspective, maybe your blood pressure goes down and your cholesterol numbers are reduced.

For many people, health and how you feel should top your list. You need to make yourself a priority. This is not an act of selfishness; this is an act of survival. It's no different than the emergency procedure on an airplane. Give yourself oxygen first and then administer it to others. The same holds true for your health. How will you be able to support and give to your family and loved ones if you are not operating at your best?

And, it's important to remember that everyone is different. Your goals are different and how your body operates is different. This is especially true as we age. What you could once do at 20 years old is radically different from what you can do at 45 years old. It's a battle against time. You need to keep your body operating as efficiently and effectively as possible.

Dominate Your Goals

There's no better time than right now to plot out your goals. When you have a clear plan of attack, it makes reaching your target that much easier.

Here are some easy-to-implement tips to help you dominate even your toughest goals:

Break Your Goal Down into Bite-Sized Segments

When you have an enormous goal like saving for a down payment on a house, running a marathon or losing 50 pounds, it's helpful to narrow down the goal to smaller steps. Look at the calendar, pick a realistic deadline and then work backwards.

Let's use losing 50 pounds as an example. A healthy rate of weight loss is 1-2 pounds per week. So, you would give yourself 30 weeks, or a little over 6 months, to lose this amount of weight. When you break a huge goal down into bite-sized segments, it becomes less scary and more attainable. Now you can break this down into 90-day, 60-day and 30-day goals. From there, you can give yourself weekly goals. Week #1 may be figuring out what diet and exercise program you will do. Week #2 may be tracking your food and establishing an exercise routine, and so on.

Write It Down

In a September 2016 article in the Huffington Post, Dr. Gail Matthews, a psychology professor at the Dominican University in California, recently studied the art and science of goal setting. She gathered 267 men and women from all over the world, and from all walks of life, including entrepreneurs, educators, healthcare professionals, artists, lawyers and bankers. Then, she divided the participants into groups, according to who wrote down their goals and dreams, and who didn't. She discovered that those who wrote down their goals and dreams on a regular basis achieved those desires at a significantly higher level than those who did not. In fact, she found that **you become 42% more likely to achieve your goals and dreams by simply writing them down on a regular basis**.

Whether you create a list of New Year's resolutions or have just one major goal to achieve, write it down in a journal, on a post-It note that you can see every day, or hang it on your refrigerator. Take it a step further and create a vision board with images of what achieving your goal will look like.

Get an Accountability Partner

Having to answer to someone can definitely put your motivation into overdrive. Do you really want to share that you haven't made any progress towards your goal? Whether you enlist a coach or a friend, you will often go above and beyond what you set out to do to prevent having to share any kind of failure or slip-ups.

How to Be Consistent

Now that you have your goals and ways to stay on track, consistency will be key to reaching them. After countless figure competitions, I know better than most people how hard it can be to stay consistent! But consistency is the key to meeting your goals. As a working mom with a side hustle, kids, a house to take care of, and a husband, life often gets in the way. It is super easy to just sit on the couch after a long day or get an extra hour and a half of sleep in the morning instead of going to the gym. Many women often tell me that they struggle with being consistent on both fronts—diet AND exercise!

Here are a few ways to help you to be more consistent:

Make It Part of Your Routine

The easiest way to remain consistent is to make fitness part of your routine, just like brushing your teeth! You don't forget to brush your teeth, right? Well, working out and eating healthy should be as much a part of your day as brushing your teeth or your hair, or taking a shower. You don't need to be at the gym for a lengthy amount of time, or spend hours of time in the kitchen creating chef-inspired healthy meals. Keep it simple and you will be more successful in your efforts!

Reward or Punish Yourself

Another great tip for remaining consistent is to either reward or punish yourself, depending on which you prefer. (Punish does not mean to deprive yourself of food!). A reward can be to get a massage or a new outfit once you reach a certain milestone. Preferably, you should stay away from food-related rewards, since using food as a reward or punishment can lead to incredibly dangerous habits and disorders surrounding food relationships. A punishment could be socking away $20-$50 dollars in savings or skipping a nail appointment. Do whatever works for you, as long as it is not food-related!

Mindset

Mindset is an area that is not frequently discussed when it comes to diet and exercise. But mindset is such a critically important component of your success! You will benefit from having the right mindset because it will help you when you're faced with making a decision to eat right or not eat right. It's also beneficial in understanding when you're full or if you're bored or thirsty. When you have the right mindset, you will be laser-focused on your goals and there won't be much that will deter you in reaching them. You've heard of the phrase "mind over matter." Your thoughts determine your actions. This is true whether your goal is to lose weight, start a business, run a marathon, or climb Mount Everest.

I never realized the importance of mindset until I started competing. I needed to be mentally prepared to dedicate time and effort to tracking what I ate. This is a different kind of rigor than working out because it's mental and it's a 24-hour commitment. Everything I put in my mouth had to be logged, because nearly everything contains calories. The foods that contain minimal to no calories can quickly add up. For example, I chew a lot of sugar-free gum, at least 4-5 pieces per day. Each piece of gum has 2 grams of carbs, so chewing 5 pieces of gum meant I was consuming 10 grams of carbs. I could've had a small rice cake!

Mindset also plays a role in self-sabotage, which is a real thing. I know because I do it to myself all the time. When I get ready for a competition and start making serious progress, I suddenly start eating outside of my prep. I know it's wrong and I know the scale will reflect it, but for some reason I don't care. I think it has to do with self-worth. Am I worthy of success? Am I worthy of coming in first place? How silly does that even sound? Of course, I am! Then why would I deliberately do things to sabotage myself? Sometimes I think we are all afraid of what will happen if we are successful, especially when it comes to losing weight. What will my friends and family think? Will people look at me differently?

The most important person you need to think about is yourself. It sounds selfish, but you have your own reasons for eating right and working out. It could be for health reasons, aesthetics, to compete, or something else altogether. Regardless, that's your motivation and that's what you need to stay focused on.

How do you improve your mindset? There are a number of ways. Read about it, understand it, learn how to improve, or even hire a coach. Some of my favorite mindset books include: *You are a Bad Ass* by Jen Sincero, *Mindset: The New Psychology of Success* by Carolyn Dweck, and *Awaken the Giant Within* by Tony Robbins. Mindset coaches are all over social media. But be sure to do your homework and understand the coach's background, methodology and outcomes. Talk to others who have successfully hired mindset coaches to guide them.

Mindset is tied closely to goals and motivation. The right frame of mind, having the confidence to achieve your goals and not letting stress or unplanned events will help keep you on track. How do you get into and remain in the right mindset? There are a few ways, and it will vary by person.

Here's the down and dirty game plan I use to work on my mindset:

SMART Goals

When you create goals, make sure they're SMART, which means Specific, Measurable, Attainable, Realistic and Timely. SMART goals are important because it makes them very precise. You will know exactly whether or not you've attained your goal. For example, if your goal is to lose weight, you would make it SMART by stating it as, "I will lose 20 pounds by May 5" or, "I will work out for 30 minutes per day, three times per week."

Affirmations

Affirmations can help you stay on track because they are a positive reminder of where your mind needs to be. No negative self-talk here. Come up with a few affirmations to help keep you on track. I have daily reminders on an app in my phone that include several affirmations:
- "My desire is stronger than my doubt."
- "Everything comes to me easily and effortlessly."
- "I deserve all of the happiness and success that I desire."

Visualization

Close your eyes and envision exactly how you want to look and feel. Picture yourself doing activities with ease, wearing clothes you've dreamed about, and feel confident and attractive.

This type of exercise is commonly used by professional athletes. Numerous studies have shown that the mental practice of focused visualization can be as effective in improving skills as real practice.

Interestingly enough, when we visualize an action – whether it's working out, sticking to our diet, getting a promoted at work – the same regions of the brain are stimulated as when we perform the action and the same neural networks are created. Essentially, your brain thinks you've already completed the task at hand!

What will it take to get you where you need to go? Start thinking about it now, not January 1. Then put a plan into place and take action. When you combine meditation, mindfulness and mindset, your goals will become easier to achieve and you will become unstoppable.

By Allison Jackson

About the author

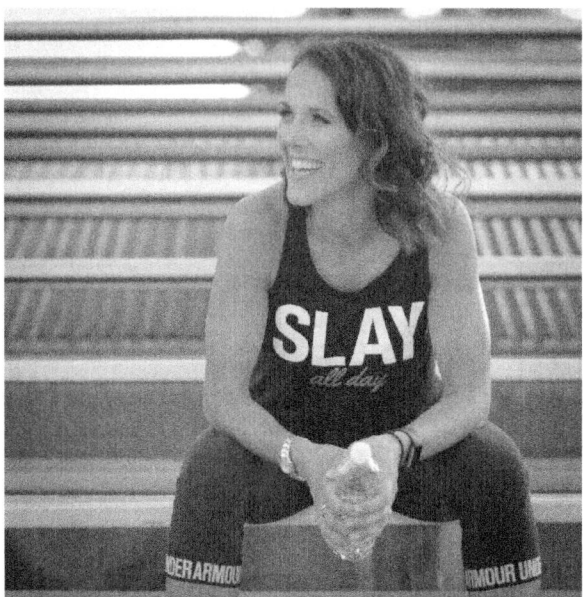

Allison Jackson is the founder of Allison Jackson Fitness, where she helps high-performing women get lean and healthy without crazy gimmicks or stress so they can lose weight and feel good in their own skin. She is a certified nutrition coach, personal trainer, yoga instructor, and pro masters figure competitor.

Allison is also a professional wellness speaker for women's retreats, trade organizations, and corporate groups. In addition to offering 1:1 and group coaching, she is also the host of the Fit to Lead podcast and author of the book Flab to Fab in 8 Weeks.

Learn more at http://www.allisonjacksonfitness.com.

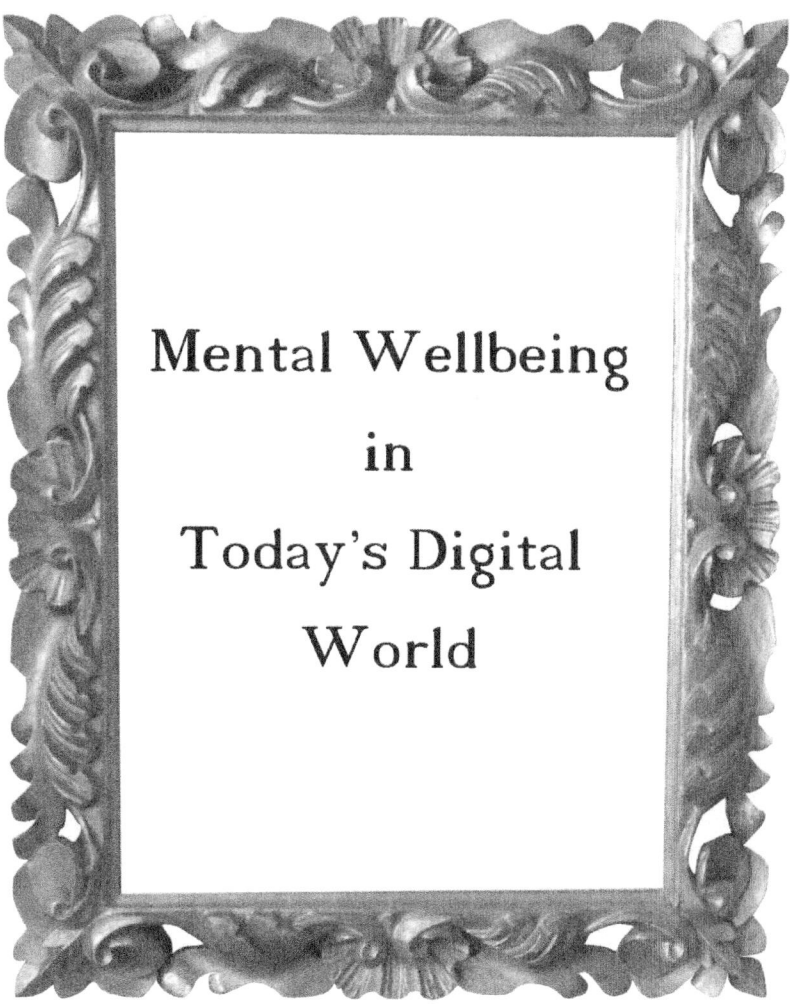

Mental Wellbeing in Today's Digital World

Mental Wellbeing in Today's Digital World

Mental wellbeing - those two words are the key to understanding everything else in our lives. Maintaining a state of wellbeing can only arise from our own thoughts, an act of conscious creation to make sure that everything is well-aligned and prevents us from experiencing burnout and mental exhaustion. The conversation around wellbeing cannot just centre around the mental and physical anymore – we need to also understand the internal, social, and digital catalysts that affect them. Our wellbeing is much more than just a state of mind and we have to be responsible for every pillar, beginning first with a solid foundation of self-understanding.

In the fast paced, consumer-driven, and overly judgmental society of today, we seem to have created a ritual for absolutely everything. Hair care, skin care, body care and more all have their own little routines and best practices. But what about mind care? When did our minds become last on the list if they're even on our lists at all? If we treat our minds with the same respect that we do in observing these other self-care rituals, we can begin to unleash its true potential – a power that can be almost like magic.

With such widespread access to the internet, social media channels, and streaming platforms, we have never before consumed so many advertisements, product placements, heavily edited photography, and other content that may not be so nourishing for our mind and soul. We must be stricter on our intake and learn to make agreements with ourselves not to get caught in the cycle of never-ending digital consumerism. That is, unless we can consciously train ourselves to focus more than half that consumption on sources of positivity, motivation, inspiration, and education.

For example, it is important to remember that social media is not real life. Every single day influencers, celebrities, and entrepreneurial users are paid to promote every type of product. From cars to holidays to watches, the people you see posting are being paid to stage and construct a certain image, and often have a professional team(s) and equipment helping them do so. These false constructions can throw off your sense of self, and make you needlessly worry about what you "should" be doing, buying, or look like. That is why it is crucial to choose the people you follow and connect with wisely. You should consciously follow people and things that make you happy, feel good, or encourage you with positivity, rather than pages that make you feel less-than or as though you need to strive for what they share on their page. More than just focusing on positive consumption, you should aim to only put out content that genuinely makes you feel good. If posting or attempting to post causes you feelings of sadness and anxiety, take a moment to think about whether it aligns with who you really are and what you want to show the world of yourself. Overall, you need to practice the use of social media with intention. Ask yourself, what do you hope to gain from your platforms that day. Is it a certain feeling, image to emulate, or status? Are you getting the results you want? If not, what do you need to change to get the right results whilst also being mindful of your true inner self?

Another often overlooked aspect of our digital world which can deeply affect your mental wellbeing is unconstrained usage. You absolutely need to set yourself times and terms of use. We can frequently fall into the trap of "doomscrolling" - staring at our feeds and wasting hours refreshing apps. Social media addiction is a very real thing and just like everything else in life we need to learn to moderate for proper usage. In fact, mapping our online consumption is a great way to organise how we spend our time, not just digitally but physically as well. Setting a weekly planner on a Sunday evening for the upcoming week and specifically scheduling in some "brain care" time can offer a reprieve from the fixed routine of scrolling through app after app, channel after channel. It is important to take a minute to reflect upon one's routine and ask, 'how is this serving me?' If you find yourself caught in a cycle which doesn't truly add value to your life or develop you in a positive way, then change must be instituted. Reviewing this monthly can ensure that we break any negative patterns that cause us to have diminished mental capacity. Conscious steps toward mental wellbeing are crucial to improving these patterns or forming new, better ones entirely.

It is important to remember that 'mental wellbeing,' or any type of wellbeing will look and feel a variety of ways to different people. There is never a 'one size fits all' solution when it comes to mental wellness. Efforts to improve your state of wellbeing should be a tailored approach toward improvement and reflect YOUR situation, mindset, emotions, energy, and spirit. Of course, the perfect state of being will never exist because in every split second our lives are forever changing. But mental wellness is not about 'perfection.' The word perfection is only held by a person's perspective of what they see, so if you invest energy in striving towards betterment, greatness is within your grasp.

You have the choice – to grow, to do better, to be better than ever before. Externally, you also have the choice to remove yourself from anything, any person or groups of people, any setting that does not fit into your route to wellbeing or positively serve you. This is called 'shedding.' It can offer a beautiful awakening on your wellness journey, but it is usually the most difficult part of the process toward mental betterment. The first step is to connect with yourself and spend time trying to identify those things and people that do not fit your future. If they feel like an obstacle to your wellbeing, then aim to initiate (at a speed/method of your comfortability) ways to spend less time engaging with these factors. Once this process begins it will be like a beacon of light shining in the darkness, showing you all that may have held you back from living your best life.

Similarly important in limiting negative aspects of your life is learning what you want to attract to it. Attracting more of what you want to become will begin to trend in your life when you are planning, prepared, and have shed the excess negatives, it allows room for more of the good, more of the positive. Abundance comes to those that have room to accept it, so we should aim to engage positive polarity in our mind. Learning to accept, attract, and adopt the positive in our lives allows for a magnetism to develop eventually and inherently pulls towards us, instead of us continuously needing to be pushed towards it.

Burnout is another important player in our mental health which is often overlooked. Even with today's increased discussion of burnout its depths and impact are still misunderstood. Burnout can be a monumental factor in our mental, physical, and emotional wellbeing. Working too much, doing too much, consuming too much, eating too much – it's as if we are always trying to outrun and out do ourselves and each other. It is time to walk and not run and attract instead of reacting. We need to finally learn that putting ourselves first isn't selfish, but necessary at times. Burnout can take us down paths to increased anxiety, sickness, and even depression. At a certain point, the option to rest will no longer be yours and your body will take over to convalesce itself where it can, even if we have not consciously prioritized it. The mind is a muscle which we are constantly exercising and straining. We would not put our bodies through the same continual process at the gym without rest in between, so the mind must be treated the same. How often we allow our minds to rest and refuel is just as vital as the way we actively use it.

Discovering our mind and developing a healthy mindset through mental exercise, rest and recovery will take some re-education and fine tuning but it's worth it. What we feed our mind ultimately affects our mood and can plant seeds of worry or doubt, so choose carefully which podcasts, books, videos, documentaries, live events, etc. you consume. Starting to adjust our mindset can be as simple as changing what we consume, shedding the negative weights, structuring our week to include rest, and updating our old routines. Eventually all the external factors which impact your mental health will align with your internal monologue and result in a higher state of consciousness and an overall elevated wellbeing.

The goal of an enlightened wellbeing will be joy. Joy is the unadulterated feeling we create when maintaining a positive wellbeing because it is not tied to anything external. Chasing external signifiers of happiness just means that your internal happiness and therefore wellbeing will be dependent on things like whether that person is happy today, whether that favoured place still exists, whether a popular item is still trending. The only thing we can control is our own attempts at joy.

There is an old adage that says, "don't pour from an empty cup, take care of yourself first" and I have always found this quote to be sending the wrong message. If you live in a way that allows your cup to be continually filled by positive manifestations, then you should instead live by the overflow system. So, never pour from your cup but instead allow your cup to be constantly filling so that you can ensure it will never be empty (and are not sacrificing your own wellbeing), but you're also allowing others to help themselves and reap the benefits of your over abundance.

The fact that you are reading this book will reinforce the journey that you are going through because your conscious choice to do so signifies your ability for growth and therefore strength. With every page and every chapter strength, confidence, and resilience will develop. In a world where it's easy to fall victim to comparison, it is important to recognise where you stand, who you are, and what you have to contribute, no matter your beginning or background. Every bit of information and interaction should act as stepping stones and bricks laid to create a solid foundation upon which to build your joyful wellbeing, to ensure its longevity and prosperity.

Simply put, your mental wellbeing is the ultimate key to a healthy and joyful existence. When we focus on our own wellbeing, it radiates to those around us and encourages a ripple effect of positive change. With a strong foundation of mental wellness, we can take on more and live a better life than ever before imaginable. As the legendary self-help author and philosopher Bob Proctor, says "if you must doubt something, doubt your limits."

By Jamie Kerr, Founder of MindKite

About the author

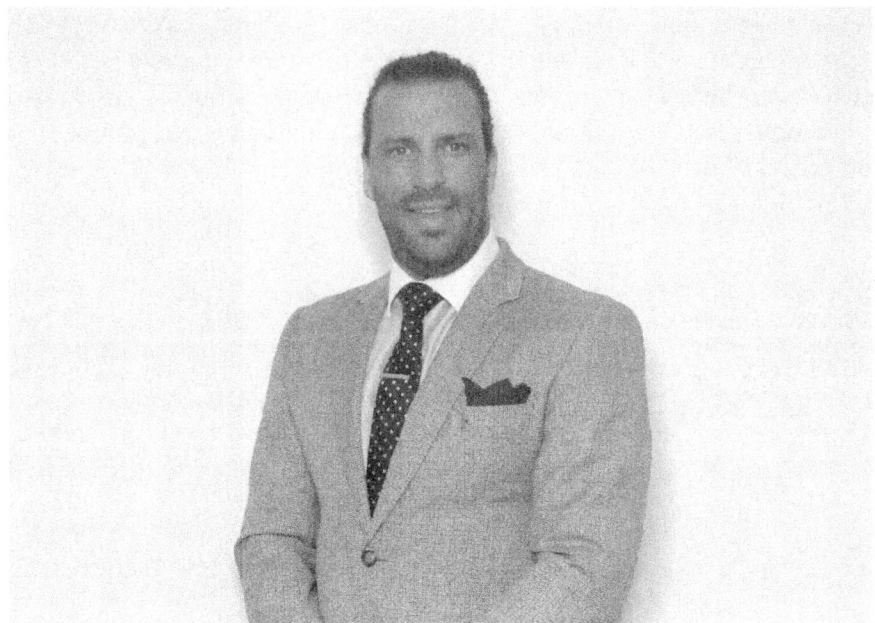

Jamie is the founder of MindKite, a mental wellbeing social media app and global community platform launched in early October 2021. MindKite's inception came with Jamie's realisation that men in his hometown of Glasgow, Scotland, were struggling with mental health, and lacked adequate support and resources. Suicide is the single biggest killer of men under 45 in the United Kingdom, with Scotland having the highest rates at 18 deaths per 100,000 persons.

MindKite aims to address mental wellbeing for men, women, teens and help to empower people through network building and social interaction, enhanced mental health literacy, and behaviour change education.

Jamie is a Performance Mentor and Mindset Coach and has spent 13 years working within psychology and mental health, dedicating his time to delivering his own unique style of mindset coaching derived from his extensive knowledge around NLP, CBT, and Life Coaching. He is also trained in Mental Health First Aid, Mental Health Awareness and holds a diploma in Psychological Coaching from the BPS-approved Centre for Coaching and a Diploma in Life Coaching

Jamie is mentored by celebrity life coach Xavier Barnett, global motivational speaker Les Brown, and internet marketing sensation Paul Getter. Jamie is also the ambassador for the charity, MindSoldiers.

Jamie has a wealth of knowledge on mental health, mindset and business, he has mentored and coached over 1000 people, racking up 20,000+ hours in assisting people to achieve, wealth, success, business growth, strengthened relationships and improved mindsets. Jamie is an expert in this industry, and can offer comments on:

- Mindfulness – the importance of positive affirmations
- Lifestyle changes – taking limiting beliefs and turning them to unlimited lives
- Social media and the impact it has on mental health
- Male suicide in Scotland and the change in mindset needed
- Suicide in the UK - breaking the pattern and noticing the signs
- Money Mindset – the impact that a lack of or too much money has on mental health/mindset

About MindKite

MindKite is a mental wellbeing social media app and platform launching early October to promote mental wellbeing, a strong mindset, safe social media use and lifestyle change. It offers its users a goals diary, positivity-driven newsfeed, global network building and social support community coupled with daily motivation and an interactive wellbeing section with custom video content. MindKite encourages reflection on how people think and talk about mental health, wellbeing and how everyone can help others to take a more positive, inclusive, and inspired use of social media.

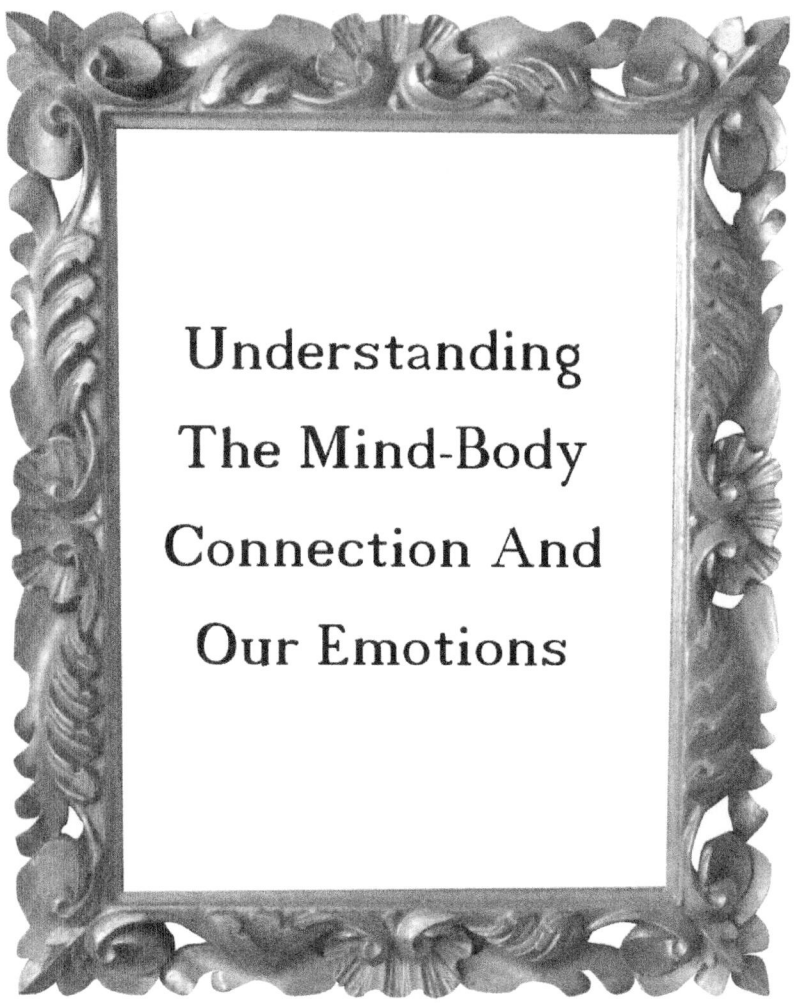

Understanding The Mind-Body Connection And Our Emotions

Understanding The Mind-Body Connection And Our Emotions

What is the mind-body connection? In short it means the belief that our thoughts, feelings, beliefs, and attitudes can positively or negatively affect our biological functioning. It is often thought that the mind and body are two separate entities, but this is not so, mental, emotional, and physical health are intertwined. Have you ever felt your stomach knot up at the thought of doing something scary? Your knees go week at the sight of blood? Smelt a certain smell when you think of a memory or person, even when said smell was nowhere around in the physical reality? Then you have experienced the mind-body connection.

The mind-body connection is not just a theory anymore with extensive research being carried out over decades by many scientists and leading experts in psychoneuroimmunology (A study of the effect of the mind on health and resistance to disease). Research has documented prolonged stress, repressed emotions and trauma alter the function of white blood cells. Stress diminishes white blood cell response to viral infections and cancer cells.

People who are more stressed are more prone to disease and infection.

Emotions and reaction

When we feel any emotion or are stressed our brain sends out thought response signals and chemicals, when faced with perceived threat or danger our body goes into flight, fight, freeze or fawn response. Our organs are programmed to respond in certain ways to situations that are viewed challenging or threatening. Cortisol (the stress hormone) is released, other functions such as digestion and the reproductive system are supressed, it alters the immune system, our sympathetic nervous system is activated (the part of our nervous system responsible for fighting off threat), the adrenal glands are activated (they are small glands which sit above the kidneys), adrenalin is also released this increases heart rate, blood pressure and blood glucose levels.
This is natural and part of human survival. But when we are exposed to long periods of stress or trauma, we are living in survival mode, and we can experience many health problems such as:
- Anxiety
- Depression
- Digestive problems
- Headaches
- Muscle tension and pain
- Heart disease, heart attack, high blood pressure or stroke
- Weight gain
- Memory and concentration impairment
- Chronic fatigue

The good news is by healing our nervous system, understanding our emotions, and working through trauma we can overcome many of these physical reactions. I will talk later about ways you can heal yourself mind, body, and spirit.

Biochemical reactions do not only occur when we are experiencing 'negative' emotions but positive ones too. It is often labelled that emotions are 'good' or 'bad' 'positive' or 'negative', I prefer to simply call them emotions; why? Because by labelling something 'bad' 'negative' our brain automatically feels like we shouldn't be feeling that way, this is where suppression or repression of emotions comes in, ignoring how you are really feeling, actively push uncomfortable thoughts, feelings, or memories out of your consciousness to avoid overwhelm, damaging your self-image or through fear. Repressed emotions are the feelings you unconsciously avoid, this will help you to forget them, but they will be stored in your subconscious and can alter your reactions and actions.

The way you deal with your emotions and stress can be a result of genetics, childhood, or life experiences, both nature and nurture are at play. Our belief systems are formed firstly in childhood with core beliefs and then more complex beliefs as we grow and experience the world around us. They are formed from a combination of biochemistry, epigenetics, learnt behaviour and environmental factors. Trauma and behaviour patterns can be passed down from generation to generation. These beliefs are how we perceive ourselves and the world around us. So can you see how our emotions and feelings have a direct effect on our bodies and health.

We have covered stress responses to emotions now let's explore the feel-good hormones.

Feel good hormones can be easily activated naturally without the use of synthetic medicines. Here are the 4 most common 'feel good chemicals';

Serotonin is the key hormone that stabilises our mood, feelings of wellbeing and happiness. It enables brain cells and other nervous system cells to communicate with each other. Serotonin also helps with sleeping, eating and digestion. To increase serotonin levels get out in the sunshine, exercise, eat certain foods and remember happy memories.

Endorphins are chemicals released by the central nervous system and pituitary gland and are linked to the opiate receptors in our brains to reduce stress and pain, they determine how we manage pain and experience pleasure. Endorphins are released during exercise, sex, eating, meditating, and laughing.

Dopamine is our reward chemical, it plays a part in how we feel pleasure, our motivation, an activity we feel as pleasurable will release dopamine, or when we complete a task, we feel good about it, this can help when we are trying to change a habit or behaviour (positive reinforcement).
Natural ways to increase dopamine production, get enough quality sleep, listen to music, eat high protein foods, meditate.
Oxytocin is a hormone that controls key aspects of the reproductive system, lactation, childbirth, and aspects of human behaviour, known as the love hormone. Ways to increase oxytocin are to have a human or animal connection, massage, social interactions with loved ones, get more vitamin D and it also said if you eat dark chocolate you can stimulate the release of oxytocin.
I hope now you are beginning to understand the importance of mind-body connection, how could they possibly be thought of as separate and how you can naturally improve your health and wellbeing by applying these concepts into your everyday life. Your mind is a powerful tool when you program it right.
I often refer to the brain as the computer system of our being, if it is full of obsessive thoughts, worry or anxiety how will it tell the rest of your body what to do clearly. By clearing the cache (a computer term for data that is automatically stored) in your brain, cleanse it of viruses and update the programming it will function more smoothly. Too much stress from current circumstances or past unhealed stress automatically running in the background will totally clog up your system. Learning stress management is a big part of improving your wellbeing.

How can the way we think affect our wellbeing?

Biochemistry is a field of science that deals with the study of chemical processes in plants and animals. Whenever you have a thought, there is a corresponding chemical reaction in your mind as a result, so how you think can affect how you feel and how you feel affects your overall health. If we change how we think, we change how we feel and as a result we can change our health and overall wellbeing. It is possible to alter the way you feel with the power of thought alone.

For example- the more you focus on illness and negativity, the more aware of that you are, the more you will attract. If you focus on pain, you will feel it. Have you heard the term 'energy flows where attention goes?' If you constantly moan, the universe will keep giving you more to moan about. If you have a positive mindset, focus on being optimistic you will attract more of this into your life. Emotions need somewhere to go, if we suppress or ignore them, they will manifest somehow at some point in the physical.

I treated a lady initially for back pain, she complained of a stabbing pain and ache in her upper back, during treatment I asked about her emotional health, she revealed someone at work had upset her, which made her angry but didn't express this in the workplace. I felt her pain was emotional rather than physical, together we explored why the situation made her feel angry and what was underneath that anger, it has triggered an emotional response in her subconscious from an old belief that she is not valued. By suppressing this emotion, it had manifested as physical pain. The lady cried as we got to the root cause and the pain diminished.

Healing the mind-body connection

I have always been very drawn to holistic health and spirituality. To me, focusing on healing just one part of who we are makes no sense for a long-term recovery, as it is a way of covering the symptoms instead of searching for the underlying causes. This is the reason in 2003 I decided to follow my passion and begin my professional journey in holistic health, spirituality, and therapeutic coaching. All focused-on mind/body connection, soul healing and overcoming trauma or illness. A concept that I work with is 'the 4 bodies and 3 minds'

The key to holistic healing is to consider a person as a whole - body, mind, emotions, and spirit. Our wellbeing, our general health depends not only on the physical, which is only one part of it, but also on our mental, emotional and spiritual bodies.

If we learn to get in touch with all four of our facets, we can begin to clear blocks we didn't know we had, heal past wounds and see our overall health improve.

The 4 bodies or planes explained:

Spiritual Body

Our spiritual body is our connection to something bigger. Whether you choose to call it the Universe / God / Source / Higher Self / Love / Life etc. really doesn't matter and would be missing the point! It is our ability to receive guidance and to surrender to something bigger than ourselves. A lot of people do not understand this and might not even acknowledge it. This aspect is not really about religion or cultural beliefs, rather about our oneness, the fact that we are all connected. This is our true essence.
Our spiritual body contains energy that it transmits to our mental body. When we are in touch with our spirituality, when our spiritual self is balanced, we tend to be calm, to not give into our fears, we feel the presence of love everywhere and trust in our higher power. We can manifest everything we need in life effortlessly.
The spiritual self is never really hurt or wounded, it is not out of balance, rather it is us that are out of alignment with it, and by being disconnected to our spirituality, we often create mental blocks (that keep the energy from flowing from the spirit to the mind).

Here's what we can do to reconnect to our essence, to the power of the Universe:
Practice meditation daily.
Work with energy clearing: Reiki, acupuncture etc.
Practice mindfulness.
Deep breathing to help us reconnect to the present moment.
Practice gratitude.
Humble the mind to the breath.
Understand that we are all one not and release all illusion of separation, comparing, judging, feeling better or less than anyone else.
Know that everything that comes our way is meant to be, is a lesson for us to learn.

Mental Body

Our mental self is formed of thoughts as well as beliefs, desires, values, goals and opinions. It is how we process information, how we learn and focus.

This mental body is formed of two parts: our little or ego-based mind and our divine mind. The egoic mind is meant to be a tool that we can use in our favour to create our own beautiful reality (setting intentions, goals, planning,). We are meant to turn it on only when we need it and then back off to live from a place of presence in the divine mind. However, this concept has been lost and we now mostly operate from our ego-based mind, which is always on and has become an incessant chatter, exhausting and loud.

When our mental self is clear and stable, when we are at peace in a state of Being, and in alignment with our divine mind, the mental body can receive the energy from the spiritual body and use it to the fullest, before it creates any form of thought.

However, when we only operate from our egoic mind, letting our thoughts rule our lives, over planning, over thinking, staying stuck in memories or in our own opinions, then we are creating mental blocks.

What we can do to heal our mental body and clear mental blocks:

Meditate (think of meditation as the path between the spiritual and the mental body - we need a clear mind to receive energy from our spiritual body)

Repeat positive affirmations. By changing the language we use to speak about ourselves and others.

Read, listen to inspirational podcasts, continue learning and expanding our mind; (I know a good one- That Inner Voice, you can find it on Amazon, Apple or Spotify)

Eliminate stress triggers.

Have and execute healthy boundaries

Emotional Body

The emotional body is the sum of all our emotional experiences. It is our nervous system, hormones, touch, water absorption and release (tears).
It is where we hold our hurtful experiences and the attached emotions and feelings like anger, sadness, jealousy, fear, guilt, resentment, shame etc. These are stored like memories in the subconscious and unconscious mind and can become emotional blocks.
Our deep wounds will typically be located at this level, in our emotional body. If we aren't aware of these emotional wounds and have not yet healed them, the negative energies they emit will influence our lives and drag us down, making us prisoners of our emotions.
Since energy flows from the mental to the emotional body, it can be blocked by emotional wounds from the past, creating anxiety, stress, more anger and all this can also impact our physical body.
Sometimes, when we react in a way we are not used to, that doesn't seem like us, the reactions are due to these emotional blocks that lie within us. We are often brought to situations and people that will trigger something inside us and open up those wounds again. This can be very painful, but it is our chance to face these wounds and to heal them.
The emotional body also stores positive feelings like abundance, love, freedom, joy etc. When we heal our emotional wounds, we are then free to enter a state of joy and love.

What helps to heal our emotional body:

Journaling: write about past experiences, childhood, and the feelings that come up.
Practice forgiving ourselves and others.
Get to the root cause of emotional blocks by seeking therapy so you can understand your emotions and release them.
Deepen our connection to others, seek to love rather than being loved, listen rather than seeking to be heard. Our presence and attention are the most precious gifts we can give to others.

Physical Body

Our physical body is the only tangible body of the four. It represents our physical experience in this lifetime, and it is through it that our spirituality, emotions, and thoughts flow. Therefore, the physical body, is a good indicator of how things are going in all areas of our life and at each level of our selves (spiritual - mental - emotional).

If we listen to our body, it will tell us if something is right or wrong. Our physical body is affected either in a healthy or in a unhealthy way by what directly goes into it (food, exercise...) but also by our thoughts and our emotions.

A balanced physical body is open, flexible, balanced, full of vitality, has all the vitamins and minerals it needs, functions well, is free of pain, is not acidic and is free of toxicity.

What we can do to take care of our physical body:

Make sure to have a good night sleep every night.
Massages, reflexology, Reiki, Acupuncture.
Exercise (running, yoga, walking, dancing)
Eat healthy balanced diet with plenty of fresh produce.
Spend time in nature; nature is so good for the soul.
Walk barefoot on the grass to ground yourself.
Learn to listen to your body, get to know it and its signs.
I have talked about the 4 bodies; I am now going to tell you about the 3 minds.
The human brain absolutely fascinates me, I remember as a kid wanting to know 'why ' all the time, why did that person do what they did etc. Human behaviour and how the body works is something I will continue to educate myself on in my practice.
When I started my NLP (Neurolinguistic Programming) coaching training in 2019, I got to delve deeper into how our brain works, especially the subconscious mind.

Conscious Mind -involves all of the things you are currently aware of thinking, short term memory and is limited in terms of capacity. Your awareness of yourself and the world around you. This is the mind of your 5 senses enabling you to experience the physical world during waking hours. By practicing mindfulness, we can live in the present moment rather than the past or future.

Subconscious Mind- is a data bank for everything which is not in your conscious mind.

It is believed the subconscious mind is responsible for over 95% of our thoughts, feelings and actions. It is where we store memories, our skills, previous experiences, everything you have seen, done, or thought, your likes and dislikes. Learning to communicate between the conscious and subconscious mind is a powerful tool on the way to success and happiness. We also store our suppressed emotions here, we run on automatic programmed behaviour, by engaging in meditation, hypnosis, or NLP sessions we can re-wired outdated beliefs, break unhelpful habits and safely replace them with relevant healthy habits and beliefs.

Super Conscious or Higher Consciousness- encompasses a higher level of awareness that sees beyond material reality and taps into the energy and consciousness behind the reality. Some refer to this as the 'ether'- the essence of the universe- a flow of electromagnetic waves that permeate all matter and space.

The superconscious is where truly great creativity is found, spiritual downloads and profound healing can happen when we tap into our superconscious minds. Deep meditation is a great way to connect with your higher consciousness. Einstein described it as 'mystic emotion' – the finest emotion of which we are capable.

You can try my 4 step AARM method I use in coaching.

A-Awareness- The first step to healing is awareness, once you become aware of how your thoughts, feelings, actions, and reactions effect your wellbeing, you can begin to make small changes every day to consciously create a happier, healthier life. How can you change what you are not aware of?

A-Acceptance- The next step is acceptance, accept that the past cannot be changed, what is, is what is! Accept where you are now is not where you will stay, everything is temporary. Practice forgiveness of yourself and others.

R- Release- Release, cry, shout, laugh- whatever comes naturally. Release what no longer serves you, people, behaviours, situations etc. Anything you also cannot change, the past, other people, the weather...you know, anything outside of you!

M-Move on- Now it is time to move on, focus on creating more love, more happy memories, live in the present moment and not be a prisoner of your past or other people.

If you would like more information on the topics, I have discussed you can reach me through my website listed below. Happy healing!

By Jennifer McKenzie

About the author

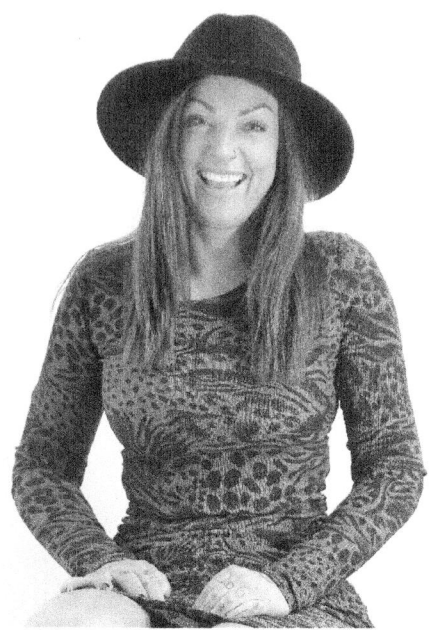

Jennifer McKenzie a 39-year-old mum of four, is a woman on a mission, living life to the full and paying forward her knowledge, expertise and life journey lessons, a life she very nearly ended on many occasions.
Now a No 1 best-selling author, host of her own wellbeing podcast, That Inner Voice, and a thriving entrepreneurial Coach with celebrity clients (The Conscious Living Coach) Jen combines her holistic therapy and spiritual experience of nearly 20 years, with her NLP life coach qualifications, bringing mindfulness into the everyday life of her clients.
Connecting science and spirituality, her work focuses on helping others to move forward in their lives from past trauma, Jen helps people to let go of their fears and stop self-sabotaging so they can live peacefully. She is also a huge body positivity activist, having learnt to love her own body after many years of being made to feel ashamed of it, working to empower other women to embrace their femininity and celebrate their bodies.
Website: www.lunarspiritwellbeing.com

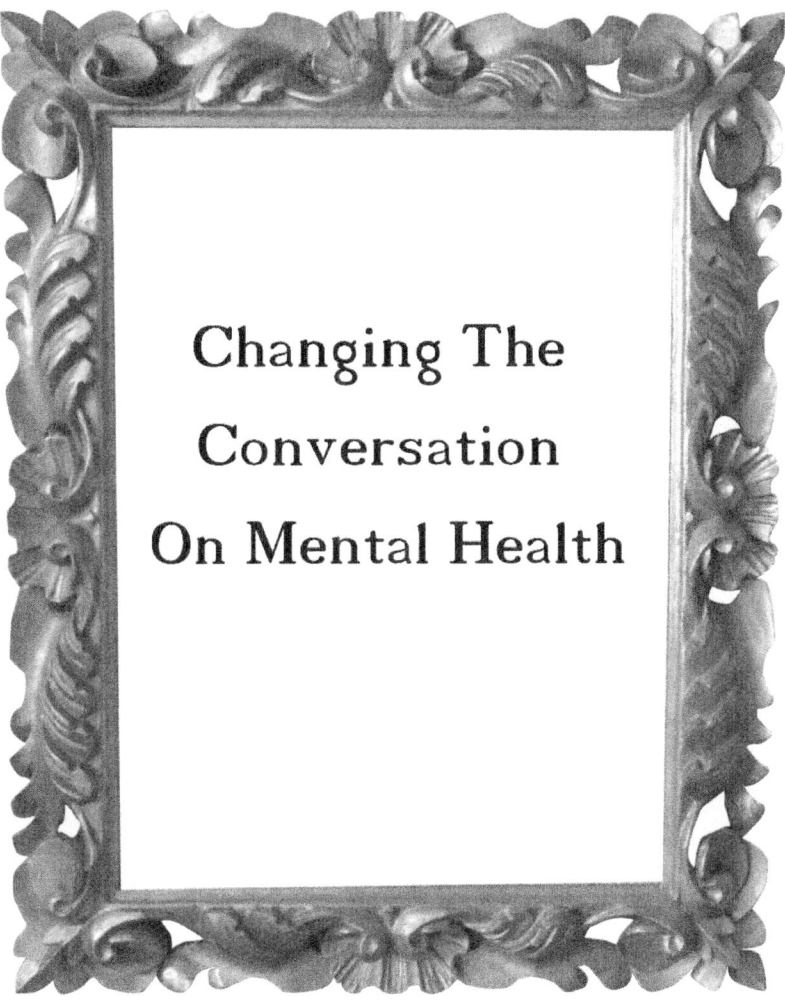

Kizzi's Health and Well-Being

Changing The Conversation On Mental Health

There can be no doubt that we have a crisis in mental health in the UK.

- During Lockdown, nearly 50% of the population were struggling with stress, anxiety and depression (PHE: Public Health England)

- Pre-lockdown only 3% of people were referred for mental health therapy (NHS 2/12/17)

- Waiting lists of 1-2 years (We Need To Talk Coalition) and even 4 years pre-lockdown

- Mental health is 13% of the NHS budget (The Centre for Economic Performance - Mental Health Policy Group, (2012). How mental illness loses out in the NHS. London School of Economics)

- In 2017, 66% of children referred for specialist mental healthcare were not receiving treatment even if they were self-harming or had suicidal thoughts. (Spurgeons children's charity)

The only realistic way out of the current mental health crisis is increasing emotional intelligence through guided self-discovery on a national scale, which means us all learning about ourselves, our minds and how we create our reality, learning to love ourselves for who we are and learning what we truly want out of life, so that we can be self-empowered to choose and then live our best life, free from debilitating stress, anxiety and depression.

The major platforms of Western society are broken, which directly or indirectly leads to mental health problems on a massive scale:

- Community, within society as a whole, has almost disappeared, with the closing of local libraries, youth hostels and playing fields. Moreover, society seems to have become more intolerant of differences, with minorities on the basis of gender and race feeling the need to demand attention; this leads to anger and anxiety. Guided self-discovery would refocus our need for togetherness: humans thrive on connection.
- The education system pressurises young people into passing exams, rather than gaining learning for life. It also completely fails to teach emotional intelligence or how to maintain one's own mental wellness...surely the most important skill for a child to leave school with in today's uncertain and complex world? A syllabus in Life Skills through guided self-discovery, including emotional intelligence, mental wellness and financial and entrepreneurial skills would correct this.
- Most business spout the phrase "our people are our biggest asset", but refuse to treat them as such, pressurising employees into longer hours, most of which are unpaid, and only retroactively signposting them for therapy once they are already struggling. They refuse to take any responsibility for the mental wellness or happiness of their staff, even though the financial benefits of doing so are enormous. Post-pandemic, employers are going to have to pay more attention to their employees' mental health, as problems are likely to be much more visible and more staff, especially millennials, are demanding more focus on the pastoral side of their work activity. Guided self-discovery on a mass scale will make this a much bigger priority in finding or changing employers.
- We have already seen the rewards of a slower, simpler life during the pandemic and lockdowns. Modern life is too fast, too stressful and too toxic and adrenaline-fueled. Guided self-discovery will allow people to explore what changes they need to make in their lives to

live that simpler, slower life. This will inevitably result in less "shopping for stuff", which in turn will dramatically reduce the ability to continue generating constant growth and force a revision to our economic model. Most importantly this will be part of the answer to reduced environmental and mental health problems.
- A more self-aware and consciously mindful population will force the politicians to change their policies and attitudes towards their electorate. Guided self-discovery will mean an electorate deeply aware of what it wants out of life and what it will demand from its government. The political status quo is not an option moving forward.

So, a widespread wave of individual guided self-discovery will, on its own, go a long way to fixing these broken elements of Western society. We have no choice, environmentally or mental health-wise, but to change the way we live and what we expect from life in order to find happiness and turn the mental health crisis around. We cannot continue to live life at 200 mph and expect our empty materialist aspirations to be fulfilled. We must learn to live a simpler, slower…and therefore more rewarding life.

But this change must come from the bottom up. We have to learn what a simpler, slower and more rewarding life means for us individually, so that we can also maximise our mental wellness. We can only do this by taking time out and going through a process of guided self-discovery. At the moment, only those who have gone through periods of significant mental illness and come out the other side, have experienced the necessary self-discovery to know what a good life for them is: and there aren't many of those. These people can be an inspiration for the rest of us, given the right community.

So, what is the journey these people have effectively been through? The rest of this chapter guides you through The Happiness Hierarchy, which constitutes our route to mental wellness. It will guide you through the journey from relatively mild stress, anxiety and depression (pretty commonplace), down into the spiral of loops of toxic thinking when left unattended and then back up through self-awareness, self-esteem, purpose, self-empowerment and finally happiness and joy.

This is a completely different way of looking at mental health. As a result, there will be a number of challenging and possibly even contentious points to be made along the way, and that needs to be the case in order to change the conversation on mental health.

Stress, Anxiety and Depression

For the vast majority of people with mental health issues, <u>mild</u> stress, anxiety and depression is the starting point. Here's the first provocative statement: stress, anxiety and depression are not mental illnesses...at least not to start with. That is how we've been taught to see them and indeed that's how we deal with them. They have a purpose, they're there for a reason. Stress, anxiety and depression are a tap on the shoulder from your system telling you your life's not working, that there's something wrong. You need to stand back, have a look and change something. We are supposed to get stressed. We're supposed to get anxious, and we're supposed to get depressed; but we're supposed to do something about them early on. The changes we need to make may be in our thinking, our behaviour, our relationships or our lifestyle. But if we treat them as mental illnesses, and we're ashamed because of the continuing stigma, we bottle our feelings up and try to ignore and avoid the signals our system is giving us. If we bottle up stress, anxiety and depression, they can only get worse, sending us into a spiral.

Fear

The problem is that underneath stress, anxiety and depression is always fear. But there are two types of fear: there is real fear, when our lives in danger, and there's false fear.

We need real fear: you're probably familiar with the fight or flight mechanism, which was literally life-saving on a daily basis for cave people millions of years ago; and yet, our system has changed much...just the world we live in. The classic illustration is as cave people, we are walking along, turn the corner and there in front of us is a sabre-toothed tiger. In an instant, all of the blood flow goes to our arms and our legs, our digestive system stops, our vision narrows and we get incredibly focussed, ready to fight or flight. Then hopefully we kill the sabre-toothed tiger or we run like crazy and we escape. Then our system comes back into balance: our heart rate slows down, our breathing slows down, and most importantly, our adrenaline levels go down, our digestion restarts, our vision widens and everything goes back to normal.

Unfortunately, false fear works in the same way. False fear is defined two words: "what if?" What if this happens? What if that happens? What if I fail my exam? What if I lose my job? These things are indeed possible, but they haven't actually happened yet: they're not real. The problem is that the unconscious mind can't tell the difference between real fear and false fear. So, your body reacts the same with false fears and worries as it does in genuine life-threatening scenarios. But unlike the sabre-toothed tiger, you can't fight or run away from losing your job or failing an exam. So, if you don't deal with what is making you anxious (even though you can't fight it or run away from it) your unconscious keeps you on "red alert", your adrenaline levels stay high and your system keeps telling you to fight or flight. Your mind is actually dealing with things as though you have failed our exam, you have lost our job, and your body is reacting that way too. You need to talk to your boss to find out how you can keep your job, you need to revise diligently for your exam, you need to deal with whatever's making you anxious. If you avoid it, the message from your system gets louder and louder, your adrenaline levels go higher and higher, your mind goes into a loop of toxic thinking, you can't sleep properly, you start making mistakes because you can't focus properly, you start upsetting people because you're getting grumpier and grumpier...you get the picture!

The additional problem we have today with regards to stress, anxiety and depression is the way we live life. We live as a constant sprint, with raised adrenaline levels keeping us going. Life is actually a marathon with... occasional sprints, but we are all running around at 200 miles an hour, going from one activity to the next, without slowing down. In cave times we weren't sat at computers all day, we were walking around constantly.

Hopefully, one of the good things that could come out of the pandemic and the lockdowns is that people have recognised the importance of slowing down, going for walk or for a bike ride, doing a bit of forest bathing. However, as things get back to normal, there are likely to be three tribes of people: those who want everything to go back to the way it was as quickly as possible; those who have recognised the importance of building me-time into their day, but unfortunately get sucked back into the constant sprint scenario and those who have learned their lesson at a deeper level, changed their lifestyle and built in downtime into each day.

Self-Doubt

So, if we bottle everything up and ignore the symptoms, the spiral starts to gather pace, and we get into self-doubt. We turn it in on ourselves, bottle everything up, blaming ourselves; we tell ourselves that nobody else has got these sorts of problems, that we're useless because we can't sort out what's going on in our heads. We doubt ourselves and start to believe that we can't sort things out.

Hiding

And then we start hiding. Now some people literally hide. In fact, scientists are expecting a wave of agoraphobia, as we come out of lockdown, people not being able to get out of their house. So, as things spiral in their heads, people start hiding, however, most of these people are actually hiding in plain sight.

I worked this out when I was still in the corporate world. I'd shut the front door in the morning and I'd already got my mask on, so that people couldn't see how "useless worthless and hopeless" I was; that's actually what I believed even though I was successfully climbing the corporate ladder. I'd got my mask on, I had a suit of armour on too to protect myself because the world's a dangerous place, especially the corporate world with people stabbing you in the back and trampling over you as they climb up the ladder. And then I had a hologram up in front of me of what I wanted people to see; this so-called better version of myself.

But behind the mask something else was going on. If I was sat in a meeting surrounded by people, I was so worried about actually asking a question and making a fool of myself and perhaps asking the wrong question, that I would actually think through the words I was going to use first before asking the question. But by the time I'd worked the words out, the conversation had moved on, and I couldn't ask the question. Then I would end up not contributing and of course beating myself up for that.

Actually, this is what virtually all of us are doing, because we're so worried about what people think about us. Most people out there in society are not being real, we've all got masks on and are pretending to be somebody else. A question for you: can you be happy being somebody else? Nope. And that's what virtually all of us are trying to do, trying to show a better version of ourselves; but it's all an act.

Self-Disdain and Self-Loathing

The problem is that behind the mask we know we're acting, and as things start to spiral it's inevitable that we go into self-disdain or even self-loathing: we start to dislike or even hate ourselves. Here's a scary statistic from the Prince's Trust's 2021 annual survey, The Youth Index: 45% of young people have been struggling with thoughts of self-loathing in the last year. That is very worrying because if you hate yourself, it completely colours how you create your reality; you are the one person you can't get away from and so you are in constant self-disdain or self-loathing and it becomes impossible to be happy: and yet this is where the spiral of stress, anxiety and depression inevitably takes you, potentially a very dark place.

So, how do we get out of the dark place?

Self-Awareness

The basic problem in mental health is that we don't know who we are: we don't have self-awareness or a sense of self. Many of my big corporate clients think they are self-aware and are somewhat offended when I say they aren't. But 91% of our mind is unconscious and therefore 91% of the way we create our reality on a moment-by-moment basis is unconscious. How much do we know about our Unconscious? Next to nothing and if we don't understand anything about our unconscious mind and the hidden programmes running in the background, then we're not self-aware.

Let me give you a personal example of an unconscious programme. I was born with very bad asthma. I was in and out of the hospital randomly, literally two or three times a month and apparently my chances of survival were only 50/50. In those days, your parents were not allowed to stay in the hospital with you. So, my parents had to constantly leave me, and apparently, if I was crying really badly, the nurses would lock me in the linen cupboard. Obviously, I don't consciously remember any of this.

Then I was packed off to boarding school at the age of seven, even though our home was only six miles away. Whilst boarding is definitely a privilege, it's not always a nice one. Because of my asthma, I was bullied constantly for two years. If you're at day school, you can come home and you're fine. At boarding school, you can't get away from it: it's 24 hours a day.

And then the Christmas at the end of that two-year period, I got mumps, and in those days that meant going to hospital and being isolated. So, I was shut away again. I still have a picture in my head of my mum in floods and floods of tears whilst my dad had to pull her away to leave the hospital.

So, what did that lead to? It was only when I trained in NLP 22 years ago that I realised I'd had an issue with abandonment most of my life. I've never actually been abandoned. But you can see when you unpack those childhood experiences, why that unconscious programming may have occurred. To make things worse, the flip side of being abandoned is that you're not worthy of love. For most of my life I did not believe I was worthy of love. But not only was this not true, I was unaware that those thoughts were going on.

We all have those sorts of programmes running in the background and they make a real difference in how we create our reality and how we feel about ourselves. True self-awareness means that we have to understand what is going on in the unconscious part of my mind; this is something that I've been teaching for 20 years. When we start to understand more about who we are and what makes us, us at a deeper level, we start to have a much better sense of identity and much deeper sense of self. This means that we are much more likely to be aware of the changes we need to make when we get stressed, anxious or depressed.

Self-Acceptance

The next step, having to learn about ourselves and who we are is to accept ourselves for who we are. We're human: we're not perfect. We mess up all the time, we tell lies, we hurt people, we do things we shouldn't do. We're not perfect. So, we need to be able to accept ourselves warts and all. When you started to unpack who you are, and you start to build a genuine, deep sense of identity, this is actually easier than you think.

Self-Esteem

The next step on the journey to mental wellness, and if ever there was a magic bullet this is it, is self-esteem. As we said earlier, if you go around hating yourself, you completely change how create your reality; your world is inevitably a much darker place. Self-esteem simply means being comfortable with who you are, being comfortable in your own skin. It is not huge levels of confidence or arrogance. In fact, contrary to how it may appear, the bully in the playground is probably the most insecure child in the school.

A lot of people in the therapy or coaching world have lots of inspirational quotes, I have one:

"Be who you are. Say what we feel. Because those who mind don't matter. And those who matter, don't mind." Dr. Seuss

When I first read that, I literally had tears in my eyes, because this is the secret to mental wellness. It is simply being comfortable with who you are...warts and all. Now, another question for you; How many people in your life do you reckon have self-esteem? How many people that you know do you reckon are comfortable in their own skin? You can't know for certain and of course there's a spectrum of self-esteem, but trust your gut and come up with an answer.

I'll tell you what the average answer is, as I've been asking people for over 15 years: on average it's between three and five. And so out of all the people we know, three to five are actually comfortable in their own skin. Okay, it's not scientific data, but how horrifying is that? We have a massive issue around self-esteem. The main reason is that we are brought up to constantly worry about what people think about us. In my day it was: "What will the neighbours think?" Who cares what the neighbours think unless they are your friends and they matter. Social media has, of course, multiplied this problem many-fold.

Here's the next serious question for you: how many people in your life actually matter? Serious question. There's your immediate family and your mates and it's not all of your mates: only the ones who would "put their lives on the line for you." If you've got more than two or three of those, you're doing pretty well. So, the average is somewhere between 12 and 15 for those who actually matter in our life. And yet we're constantly worrying about what everybody thinks about us all the time, because we've been brought up to do it. And actually, virtually nobody matters.

Here's a challenge for you: give me one good reason why you shouldn't be comfortable with who you are. Yes, we've all failed at something, hurt those we love and done things we regret. But that doesn't mean to say that we can't be comfortable with who we are. In fact, if we want to be successful, live a good life and create loving relationships, it's essential that we're comfortable with who we are. So, give me one good reason that stands up, as to why you shouldn't be comfortable with who you are. In 15 plus years of challenging people on this, I've never been given one good reason.

This is not about being arrogant or over-confident, it just means that we need to stop being worried about what people think about us. Worrying about what people think relates directly to lack of self-esteem and self-loathing. It is a massive issue in society today. Gathering self-esteem may sound like a mountain that you have to climb, but when you have built a reasonable sense of identity, you're already half way to being comfortable with who you are. Having self-esteem is not difficult, but it is the key to mental wellness and living a good life. Self-esteem gives your life a positive glow in terms of how you create it, consciously and unconsciously, rather than the grey clouds generated by self-loathing.

Authenticity

The next step up from self-esteem is authenticity. This means that when you've started to feel comfortable with who you are, you've got to go out into the world and be that person: be you...no mask, no armour, no hologram. That might sound scary, but you as you go through the journey of self-awareness, self-acceptance, and self-esteem, it is not as difficult as you think. Because when you stop worrying about what everybody thinks about you, you don't need the mask.

In order to drop the mask, you've got to be prepared to be vulnerable. However, we've been taught not to be vulnerable, particularly in our work environment. In fact, as kids we're brought up to actually hide our weaknesses. And yet, showing our weaknesses and being vulnerable in is the most powerful thing in the world; it's charismatic. That doesn't seem to make any sense; it's counter-intuitive. In fact, any person in any field of human activity that stands head and shoulders above the others, is being vulnerable: they are showing their weaknesses. It's just that we don't see it. So, let me give you some examples. Sir Richard Branson is dyslexic and has been supporting charities for dyslexia for 45 years. At school he was told he was thick, because at that time we didn't know what dyslexia was. As soon as he was diagnosed, he came out and told everybody, he set up a charity. He has never hidden the fact that he is dyslexic, and it has not stopped him being one of the most successful entrepreneurs in the world. So, is Richard Branson, weak and vulnerable? No.

It was Sir Winston Churchill who came up with the expression of "the black dog with depression". In other words, the whole electorate knew that he was depressed. Was Winston Churchill weak and vulnerable? No.
By all accounts Adele is a very private person but she's very open about mental health issues. She is also responsible for the single most authentic piece of live TV I've ever seen. She was doing a tribute to George Michael with a 50-piece orchestra behind her. They start playing, she starts singing and then about four or five seconds later she says: "Stop! Stop! I've completely messed that up. Can we start again please?" That is staggering authenticity. Is that weak and vulnerable? No!
Another of my heroes is Olly Alexander. He's the lead singer of Years and Years, a successful pop band. He was also in the TV programme "It's a Sin" about AIDS in the 1980s. He is openly gay and openly talks about his mental health issues. Is he weak and vulnerable? No!
These guys are heroes because they're actually out there talking about their weaknesses or rather what elements of the public will see as weaknesses. They are not hiding. They are being vulnerable. And yet, we don't see any of those people as weak, but as charismatic. So, simply going out into the world as yourself without a mask is charismatic. When I understood the power of this 15 years ago, I put up on my website home page that I'd had a breakdown. I'm not ashamed of it; it's just what happened in my life and I'm happy to share it. When you're no longer hiding in plain sight, you can be happy.
The reason I think this is charismatic is not obvious: it's to do with the way we communicate as human beings. There is some disagreement scientifically to the exact breakdown but it is commonly agreed that 7% of the way we communicate is in the language or the words we use. 38% is in the tonality: the way we deliver the words, which includes hand gestures. So, for example, if somebody is shouting their head off at you, you don't even hear what they're saying, you pay attention to the anger, and the way they're delivering the message.
But that leaves 55%. 55% of human communication is completely unconscious, we don't know how we do it. Now, the nearest most people have experienced this, is when you meet somebody for the first time, you shake hands, look in their eyes, smile, and you know you like that person. How do you know that? They haven't said anything yet. That's the unconscious communication. So how does that work?

It might not be the mainstream view but that unconscious communication must be energetic. Obviously, we have energy pulsing through our body and your physics teacher would have told you that any energy has a field. You may remember playing with iron filings and a magnet; that's an example of an energy field. In other words, human beings have an energy field and the average energy field goes out about 10 feet from our body. So, when you're shaking somebody's hand, you're sufficiently physically close that your energy fields are overlapping. That means our feelings are able to pick things up energetically from the other person and this is a large part of our unconscious communication.

If somebody has got a mask and hologram up, there's effectively an invisible barrier in the energy field between them and the person they're talking to. We are very adept at picking up unconscious signals from other people; we know when somebody is not being open, honest or authentic: we pick it up unconsciously. So, when somebody does not have a mask on or hologram up, there's no barrier. Their communication is more authentic, more true, more open. And you can only do that if you're not hiding your weaknesses. So those people who are charismatic are not worried about what people think about them: they're not hiding and 100% of their communication is saying the same thing and that is very unusual. This is why showing your weaknesses is the most charismatic thing in the world.

Life Purpose

The next step to happiness is having a life purpose. If you'd have asked me 20 years ago what I wanted out of life, it was simple: money. And in fact, if you ask most adults, what they want out of life, 9 times out of 10, the answer will be something around financial security. I understand that. But what else? Most people don't know; they don't really know what they want out of life. The way we seek happiness is that we seek it outside of us: we go out for a meal, we got the cinema, we go on holiday. It is critical, now more than ever, that kids leave school knowing what they want out of life.

I had to have a breakdown to find out what my purpose was. I actually believe every single one of us has a purpose, but we have to look for it. It doesn't mean to say that everybody has to train as a therapist or a teacher. This is the reason that 80% of the UK workforce is disengaged from their work. In other words, they spend 65+% of their waking life doing something they don't enjoy. Our work has to be something that makes us happy, rather than just waiting for a cheque to pay the bills.

Actually, what we're really after is joy, rather than happiness. It might sound like I'm playing with words, but joy is different to happiness: it's inside of us. To have joy you need a good sense of self, you've need to have accepted who you are, warts and all, you need to be comfortable in your own skin, you've got to go out into the world, with no mask, no hologram, and you've got to know what you want out of life.

Self-Empowerment

This self-discovery work is not only simple, but fascinating. The journey of self-discovery from self-awareness, through self-esteem, authenticity and life purpose is extremely empowering. Not only do we immediately listen to our systems when they tell us that something's wrong (we're just starting to get a little stressed, anxious or depressed) and make changes in our lives, ensuring that we stay mentally well, but we thrive by living the life we choose.

Individual self-discovery is so much more than mental wellness; if we followed the path collectively, it would transform community and society, giving us the understanding and passion to demand changes in the education, medical, business and capitalist structures in the Western world.

By Mark Newey: Protagonist, Teacher, Maverick

About the author

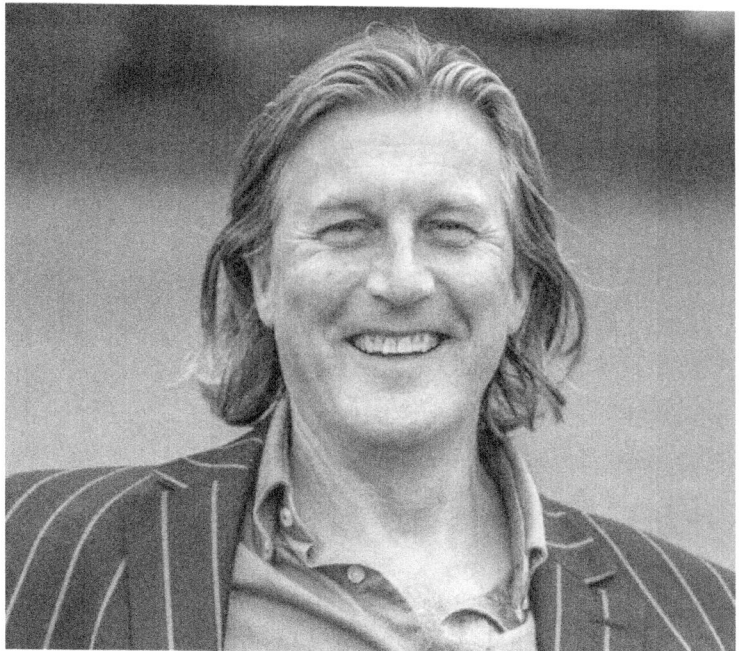

Mission

To change the conversation on mental health and transform the nation's mental wellness through Therapeutic Self Discovery.

Training and Experience

After 18 extremely stressful years of working for huge corporations in international marketing, Mark had a breakdown in 1999. Rather than going on medication, Mark fought through his breakdown, creating a huge curiosity in the mind.
This led to him training in the neurosciences and a complete career change, as a Mental Wellness Coach and Teacher, becoming his life's work and calling. Over the last 20 years he has helped thousands of people, from

school children through to top corporate directors, to beat Stress, Anxiety and Depression.

He is now bringing his unique knowledge and understanding of mental health issues to a much wider audience through speaking engagements, seminars and workshops for companies and individuals and an online mental wellness platform.

The current reactive approach to mental health is broken and disempowering. We must change our approach and employers will be key to heading off what could be a national disaster.

mark@headucate.me

www.headucate.me

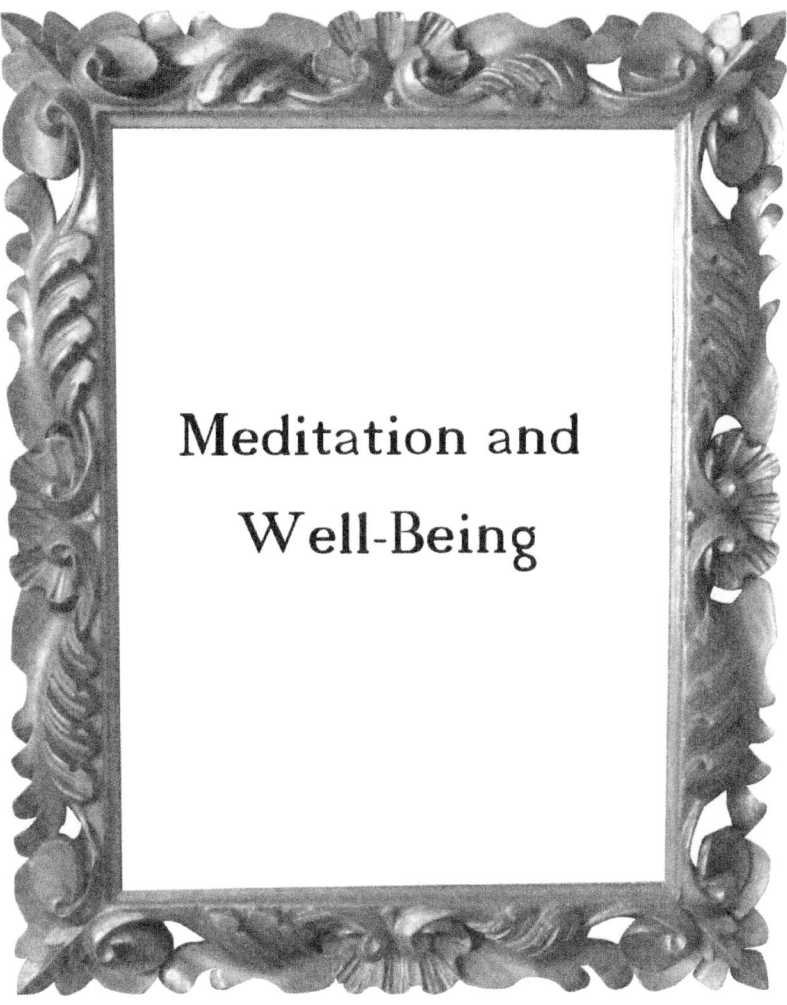

Meditation and Well-Being

Meditation and Well-Being

The practice of meditation is still shrouded by mystery, and for many, there is confusion as to what it's actually all about. I think the reason for this is that everyone's meditation experience is unique and deeply personal. In essence, meditation is the practice of focussing one's mind to become aware of what is going on within and around oneself.

There are many different techniques and purposes for meditating. While it was once more exclusively practiced in religious traditions by those seeking spiritual enlightenment, meditation has become mainstream, being practiced by people from all walks of life.

The rising popularity is no doubt due to the many benefits of this ancient practice, especially as it promotes inner and outer wellbeing. Best of all, it's a natural and simple process accessible to everyone. Given our fast pace lifestyles and the chaotic world that we live in, it's never been more important to be able to connect with the inner calm that resides at the centre of our being.

I believe it is the most inspiring, powerful and life enhancing practice to incorporate in one's life. So let's explore what meditation is about.

My Personal Journey

I remember the first time I did a formal meditation as if it were yesterday. At the time I had no understanding of what meditation was, nor did any of my school friends. We scoffed at the idea of sitting in the hall with our eyes closed on a Friday afternoon. It seemed like we were being punished, having to endure what we imagined would be an hour of boredom.

The meditation teacher took us through a guided visualisation journey. At first there were lots of giggles in the room, but soon everyone had settled down, and before long I drifted into a state of deep relaxation. I could actually feel my mind opening up to an altered state. It was as though I was travelling through space and time. I'd lost all sense that I was lying down in the school hall and was surrounded by thirty other students. When my attention was brought back into the room, I knew that this was something that I wanted to do more of. Not everyone else felt the same way about it. Some of the girls couldn't get into it at all, others found it mildly relaxing, while for me it was life changing. What I experienced reminded me of how I used to feel as a small child when I spent hours in the garden creating fantastical worlds in my mind and embarked on grand adventures of my own imaginings. My mind was free to roam and explore, there were no rules and no limits. I just wasn't allowed to leave the backyard.

From that day on, with the little I knew about meditation, I would use my imagination to take me on journeys of my own creation. I wasn't doing it to achieve any particular outcome. I just really enjoyed experiencing the different sensations and feelings of freedom that accompanied it. My mind was free to roam to wherever it wanted to go, completely uninhibited and unrestricted. I didn't think about whether I was doing it right or wrong, and in fact, I don't even think I recognised that what I was doing was a form of meditation, it just felt good to let my imagination run free. In my mind, I would soar across the sky, explore jungles, drift in rafts, visit ancient cities, fly on a magic carpet, or just allow whatever came into my mind to present itself. This became part of my evening routine, and I would usually fall asleep during the experience.

I loved diving into my mind and was curious about the different emotional states that I was capable of evoking, even though at the time, I didn't understand what I was doing. At some point in my late teens I became distracted by the adventures of life and forgot all about my mind journeys. In my mid-twenties, I became very ill, and during this time I began to re-evaluate what life was about and the search for something more commenced. It was at this point that I joined a group which practiced guided visualisation techniques, which I still find to be one of my favourite meditation styles. Over the years, I've practiced a number of meditation styles and run meditation workshops.

I've witnessed profound changes occur when people incorporate a meditation practice into their lives. It is like a key that unlocks a doorway to the innermost aspects of ones being, providing a deeper dimension to the quality of life and overall wellbeing.

My meditation practice has supported and enhanced my life in many different ways. I meditate for relaxation, mental clarity, to manage my emotions, to seek guidance, to connect more deeply with myself, to shift perspective, to fall asleep, to inspire creativity, to feel more energised, for spiritual transcendence, and so much more. It is an ever evolving part of my life that allows me to detach from the distractions and noise of this world and to connect with a deep sense of inner peace and love. If I happen to not meditate for some particular reason, I really notice the difference it makes to my state of mind. I'm passionate about the benefits of meditation and its importance to maintaining a healthy and balanced lifestyle, particularly given the fast pace world that we live in. While the technique is simple, the benefits are profound. Its simplicity belies the enormity of the gifts it has to offer.

What Is Meditation?

"What lies behind us and what lies before us are tiny matters compared to what lies within us", Ralph Waldo Emerson

Meditation is essentially the practice of focussing one's mind. Webster's dictionary defines the term "to meditate" as "to engage in thought or contemplation; reflect". People often say that they find meditation difficult as they can't get their mind to stop thinking. Our minds are designed to think, meditation is not an attempt to stop the mind from thinking. It is, however, a technique of focussing and redirecting ones thoughts. Thoughts are very powerful things! The quality of our thoughts determines the quality of our lives, and what is most interesting of all is that for the most part, we are unaware of what is going on in our heads.

I have heard someone liken the mind to a wild horse, which I think is wonderful metaphor. Without taming it, it will take you wherever it will. By taking the time to tame, nurture and care for the horse, you then become the master of your journey, as you are the one deciding on the course of direction with a trusted friend, rather than your mind taking you on a wild ride with no destination. We want our mind to be our trusted friend not our foe. Our unchecked thoughts are often our greatest enemy, preventing us from achieving and living a fulfilled life. Meditation is a way of taming, nurturing and caring for the mind so that we can clearly direct our thoughts to improve our wellbeing and quality of life.

Consider the fact that where your mind goes, energy follows. Your thoughts influence the way you feel, the way you feel colours your perception of yourself and the world around you, which determines your experiences and the way you engage (or disengage) with life, which further reinforces the way you think, which determines the way you feel…As you can see, it becomes a loop. The more you think and feel the same thoughts and emotions, the more you become those thoughts and emotions.

This reinforces the concept that you are what you think. The practice of meditation is based on the principle that "energy follows thought". It all starts in your head, so it makes sense to be aware of what is going on in your head, as by doing so, you gain greater mastery over your life. In order to have mastery of your life, you must be the master of your mind. Meditation is a discipline that enables you to achieve such mastery which is why it is a practice that is also used by professional athletes. By repeatedly imaging a desired outcome, their performance is enhanced. Such is the power of the mind.

Our mind, body and soul are intrinsically connected. While we experience thoughts and feelings, we are not our thoughts or our feelings. Our thoughts can be changed, as to can our emotions. Even if you change your thoughts and emotions, you are still essentially you, but with a different outlook or mindset. This is what the science of meditation is based on. By redirecting your thoughts, you redirect your emotions, which shifts your mindset, influencing your experience and quality of life. And it doesn't necessarily have to happen in that order.

The physical, mental, emotional and spiritual aspects of our being are intertwined. If there is an imbalance in one aspect of our being, our entire being is impacted as the overall flow of energy through our system is affected. For example, if you are experiencing physical pain, you are not likely to be in the best of moods. The physical pain, or imbalance, also impacts your emotional and mental state of being. As is the case when somebody is delivered bad news. Not only do they have an emotional and mental reaction, but often there is also a physical reaction to the information.

When people feel stressed, it is common that they experience the stress in their bodies as physical tension, particularly in their neck and shoulders. If they take the time to get a massage, not only do they experience physical relaxation but they tend to feel emotionally lighter and mentally clearer. People exercise not only as it improves their physical health, they also experience mental clarity and a sense of feeling good. These examples show the relationship between the mind, body and emotions.

So if we are not our thoughts or our feelings, who are we? Beyond our thoughts, our emotions and our bodies, there is our higher mind. It is the pure essence of our being, the truth of who we are. In different teachings, the higher mind is described in many different terms, such as the essential self, authentic self, soul self, higher self, conscious self, whole self, pure self, eternal self and so on. During the process of meditation, we are directing our thoughts from our lower mind to our higher mind, from a lower awareness to a higher awareness. This gives us the opportunity to free ourselves from the mental loops of the lower mind that we tend to get caught up in. The lower mind is often referred to as the concrete mind. It is rational, logical, linear, analytical and factual by nature, its focus planted on the material reality and survival. The lower mind is also critical, judgmental, automatic, limiting and habitual. Most of the time, we are using our lower mind. The higher mind is creative, intuitive, abstract and infinite by nature. It is from the higher mind that we experience inspiration, creativity, new ideas, and higher consciousness. Your higher mind determines your personal experience and quality of life.

Our minds get caught in mental loops. Studies show that the average mind has between 25,000 to 50,000 thoughts a day. Some sources claim a much greater figure, while others indicate that it is far less than this. Whatever the amount, it's a lot of thinking. What is of interest here, is that according to some research, 98 percent of our thoughts are exactly the same as the same as the ones we had the day before. This shows us that we truly are creatures of habit. What we are worried about today is most likely what we were worried about yesterday, last week, last year or perhaps even last decade. Our minds get caught up in mental loops, so much so that we are unaware of what we are thinking. Some of this may be to our advantage, in that it is time saving. We don't have to think about what we're doing, we just do it out of habit. We are running on auto-pilot. For instance, we tend to go to sleep on the same side of the bed, wake up to the same morning routine, eat the same breakfast, hold our toothbrush with the same hand, take the same route to work, go to the same place to get lunch, talk to the same people, have the same conversations, and so it goes. Our lives are predictable because we keep living from the same thought processes. There is nothing particularly wrong with this, however it highlights that we aren't necessarily conscious of what we are doing. For a big part of our day, we are doing things unconsciously.

By thinking the same thoughts, we keep recreating the same life experiences. Living this way may offer us a level of comfort, but it can keep us stuck in mindsets that limit our experiences and restrict our opportunity to live a more fulfilled life. For many, their "comfort zone" can actually be very uncomfortable. I call this living in the "comfortable uncomfortable".

As much as we like to complain about our life circumstances, most of us prefer to stay in the comfort of our discomfort rather than seek change. Even if we were to change our external situation, that doesn't necessarily mean that we will feel anymore joy, satisfaction or peace of mind. For instance, if someone suffers from anxiety, the anxiety isn't going to go away simply because they move into a new house.

The anxiety lives within them, it's going to follow them along with the move. Essentially, wherever you go, there you are. Real change begins from within, and that's what a meditation process is all about. It's an inside job.

By becoming aware of what is going on within us, we have the ability to consciously redirect our thoughts, emotions and overall mindset so that we are better equipped to deal with the world at large. We are likely to make better choices when we are have a relaxed and composed state of mind, as opposed to when we are feeling anxious, stressed or nervous. Meditation offers the ability to shift our inner state of being, that is the gift of this ancient tradition.

Regardless of what is happening in our external environment, we are not at the mercy of those conditions to dictate how we think or feel. Rather than being reactive, we become responsive.

Meditation isn't going to make all of the bad things in life go away, but it certainly helps to create a solid inner foundation so that we have greater mastery in navigating our way through life. That is why it is so passionately promoted by those that practice it. A friend of mine has recently taken up meditation and she can't believe the difference it has made in her life. She has been experiencing some major upheaval which has taken her on an emotional and mental roller coaster. While there is still a great deal of uncertainty all around her, her meditation practice has given her a sense of inner peace and calm which will no doubt enable her to move through this phase more gently. Her whole demeanour has changed simply by including twenty minutes of meditation a day. I can now see the light in her eyes which was has not been there for quite some time. She feels like she's discovered some great secret, even though I've been encouraging her to try it for years.

Meditation is a way of keeping the mind fit and agile, and we all know how important our mental fitness is in life. Within our minds is infinite possibility, yet we mostly live in the same tiny little garden patch of this infinite field of potential. Meditation helps us to move beyond our limitations, opening us up to our greater potential. It helps us to break out of the mental loops of our lower mind and opens us to new ways of thinking and being. If you want to change the way you feel, start by changing the quality of your thoughts. To change the quality of your thoughts, first you need to become more aware of your thoughts.

Meditation is a technique of bringing your awareness to your thoughts, which enables you to redirect your thoughts and also move beyond your thoughts. The experience of "beyond" is a deeply relaxed meditative state of heightened awareness. People experience and describe it in many different ways, however I don't think words can provide an accurate description of this state of blissful peace. This heightened state of awareness is not always achieved in meditation, but that does not mean that the meditation is less effective. Even two minutes of focussing on your breathing can effectively reduce stress levels and help clear your mind.

While it is a simple process, it can take time to master the art of meditation. It's not something you get right or wrong, it's an ongoing and evolving process. From an early age, we are taught to care for our physical bodies. We eat, bathe, groom, exercise, nurture, medicate, and take care of the needs of our body, but in general, we are not taught to do the same for our minds. When you think about it, this is rather strange, given that the health of our mind very much determines our overall wellbeing.

A miserable mind creates a miserable life, while a joyous mind is conducive to a joyous life. The practice of meditation is regarded as medicine for the mind. By meditating, we are active participants in our wellbeing. Focussing the mind on the present allows one to let go of the worries from the past and release the fears of the future. This gives the mind the space it needs to breathe, realign and recalibrate. Think of it as a short holiday for the mind. We all know the benefits of taking time out to go on vacation. Stepping out of our monotonous routines gives us the time to refresh, renew, and gain a new perspective. This is what happens during meditation, without the expense or need to pack a travel bag!

Why It Is More Important Than Ever To Meditate

There is no doubt that we are living in a fast pace world that can impact our wellbeing in an adverse way. Technology has connected us to the world in a way that we have never been before. The world is now at our fingertips and in the western world it is hard to find an adult that does not own a mobile phone. We are posting, liking, commenting, swiping, googling, texting, snap chatting, Instagramming, shopping, banking, etcetera, without having to leave the house. And when we do leave the house, our precious devices come with us so we don't have to miss out on anything that is going on. Unless we make a conscious effort to switch off, we are always on. While technology benefits our lives in many ways, we are seeing the negative ramifications of how it is impacting our lives. To name a few examples, there is young children addicted to their devices, cyberbullying, anxieties being fuelled as people compare their lives to the happy perfect images they see on their screen, people not a hundred percent present as they are constantly distracted by their phone, and technology replacing people's jobs, in turn reducing the need for any real social interaction. The list goes on.

With the constant distraction, people's attention is flitting from one thing to another. At this point in time, we may not be fully aware of what the long term consequences of the use of technology may be. I personally believe that it is more important now than ever to be able to switch off and take care of our inner needs. Without doing so, we're not giving our minds the space to relax, take stock and breathe. Not only are people dealing with influences of rapid technological advancements, but we are also exposed to global events that are creating a sense of unease. Frequent headlines of terrorism, global warming, financial crisis, natural disasters, unstable political environments, superbugs, and social struggles bombard us. These are a stark contrast to the images of the glamorous lifestyles of the rich and famous that our society worships. It is little wonder that mental health issues are such a problem in our culture.

Having a meditation practice assists in promoting and maintaining mental and emotional health. It is a way of moving beyond all the external noise and distractions to connect with the inner calm that resides within us. Living in rapidly changing times means that we too must change with the times. This can be very overwhelming, stressful, exhausting and confusing. We are living in a time when we are so connected by technology yet so many people are feeling lonely and disconnected from the community.

We spend the majority of our time focussed on what's going on around us with little regard to paying attention to what's going on within us. There is a prevalent belief that the solutions to our problems are out there somewhere. The underlying philosophy of meditation is that the solutions reside within us. Considering that what's going on in our heads drastically impacts the way we engage with the world and the quality of our lives, it makes natural sense to prioritise and care for our minds. Meditation is a way of becoming more consciously aware, allowing us to deeply connect with ourselves so that we may actively observe and transform our state of being. Being able to connect with feelings of inner peace, calm and joy goes a long way in cultivating a dynamic and fulfilling life. The power truly is within each of us, and meditation is a natural and gentle way of tapping into that.

Don't Give Up

Most people give up after only a couple of attempts of meditation. While it is a simple process, it can be difficult to get into at first. That's because we are not taught to sit with ourselves in silence. We live in a very mentally active culture, where our minds are always switched on. Our first attempts to meditate can feel very unnatural and even uncomfortable because our minds are likely to be telling us that we should be doing something. Sitting down may feel like a waste of time and you may not even be sure of what to expect. I think it's important to go into meditation with a spirit of openness. Think of it as an experiment and allow the experience to unfold as it will. With time and practice the benefits will be revealed.

When I have taught and participated in group meditations, I've found that everyone's experiences are different even though they have all been guided through the same process. That is the beautiful aspect of meditation, there are no limits as to what may unfold. It's a path of self-understanding and self-discovery which is available to everyone, any time, at any stage of life. It's easy to become frustrated when learning to meditate as we tend to expect immediate results, and many people do experience immediate results. But if you're not one of those people, keep trying. Try not to think of it as chore or as something you have to do. Think of it as a time to just sit and relax.

Meditation takes time. The more you practice it, the easier it becomes. Don't give up, even if your lower mind attempts to convince you of a million different reasons not to bother with it. Remember, the lower mind is practical, logical and often critical and it is likely to tell you that you are wasting your time and that there are more fun things for you to be doing than sitting there with your eyes closed. The lower mind has been running the show for a long time, so it's not going to let go of its rulership without a fight! As you shift your awareness to your higher mind, your perception is altered to a higher awareness. This shift, even if minor, changes the way you think, and as a result your personal experiences and quality of life are transformed. Be patient with it, as it is a practice which can add deeper and richer dimensions to your life and improve your overall wellbeing. As with any practice, the more you put into it the more you'll get out of it, and this is certainly the case with meditation.

There really is no getting it right or wrong. Make the time to take as little as five minutes a day to meditate. You may want to try a few different meditation techniques before finding the one that works best for you. Even seasoned meditators experience periods where they find it difficult to get into a meditative zone.

Another thing that tends to happen when people first start meditating is that they fall asleep. Unless you are meditating to help you fall asleep, it's not a good idea to do it lying down as the chances are you'll be asleep in no time. It's best practiced sitting up with your spine straight and relaxed. You may be falling asleep because you're tired, so as soon as you begin to drift into relaxation you'll nod off. This is very common and it's okay. Sometimes you may actually feel like you've fallen asleep but you have in fact experienced a state of deep relaxation. Keep at it, and with time you'll become more alert and aware during your practice.

While there are many books and literature on the topic of meditation, it is best to experience it rather than to read about it.

Where And When To Mediate

It's best to meditate in a quiet place where you won't be interrupted. Meditating in bed is not recommended, unless you want to fall asleep, as your body associates your bed as a place to sleep.

Some people like to create a sacred space for their meditation practice and create a ritual for this special time. I enjoy meditating in nature but really anywhere is possible.

You can meditate at any time of the day, however it is recommended that you meditate in the morning before the mind gets too busy. A morning meditation is great way to set yourself up to have the best day possible.

Types Of Meditation

There are many different types of meditation. It's about finding the right style of meditation that works best for you and that may change and evolve for you over time. Sometimes we naturally achieve a meditative state when we are really engaged in an activity, such as painting, surfing, gardening, exercising or when we are just sitting down watching the world go by. Following are some popular meditation types to name a few, but there are many more.

Guided visualisation meditation is a popular form of meditation as it gives the mind something to focus on. It engages the power of the imagination to evoke positive feelings including relaxation and stress relief. There are numerous guided visualisation meditations to choose from depending on what your needs are.

Mindfulness meditation is about bringing ones full awareness to the present moment and simply observing without judgement. This meditation can be done anywhere. Loving-kindness meditation (Metta meditation) promotes feelings of compassion and love for others and for oneself.

Vipassana Meditation is an ancient Indian meditation technique which is usually taught in a course over a number of days. The objective of Vipassana is self-transformation through self-observation.

Transcendental meditation focusses on the repetition of a single mantra. This technique promotes a deep state of relaxation and inner peace with the main purpose to reach the state of enlightenment.

Body scan meditation uses the technique of scanning the body from head to toe and identify areas of tension. The aim is then to release the tension in order to experience deep relaxation.

Zen meditation is usually practices in Zen Buddhist centres with an emphasis on correct posture. Yoga Meditation involves performing a series of postures and controlled breathing which helps calm the mind.

Qi Gong focuses on breathing techniques, movement and meditation to promote wellness.

Benefits Of Meditation

Regardless of which type of meditation you choose to do, I think one of the greatest benefits of meditation is the very act of taking some time out to spend time with yourself. Creating the space to focus on your mental, emotional and physical health goes a long way to your overall wellbeing. Meditation is a very nurturing practice and a form of self-care. The greatest healer resides within oneself and meditation is often described as medicine for the mind. When the going gets tough, get meditating and get meditating so it's not so tough going! There is no doubt that we are living in a very chaotic world. If you are looking to find a sense of inner peace, to reduce stress, to experience more positive emotions, to find clarity and purpose, to feel more energised, improve overall wellbeing, promote healing, feel more inspired, slow the aging process, experience greater inner harmony, meditation is the path to consider.

I've referred to meditation as a practice, technique, medicine, science, and an art. It is indeed all of these things, yet it is so much more. There are worlds to be discovered within you that you cannot even imagine and meditation provides the key to accessing these worlds. It is a way of life that is deeply enriching, and this is the reason that this ancient tradition is still thriving today. Our wellness starts from within. In these chaotic, stressful and turbulent times, it has never been more essential to our wellbeing to find a place of inner calm. Meditation is a natural and practical way of maintaining and igniting our wellbeing. I sincerely hope you that you feel inspired to explore this sacred art.

By Rosemary Sherro

About the author

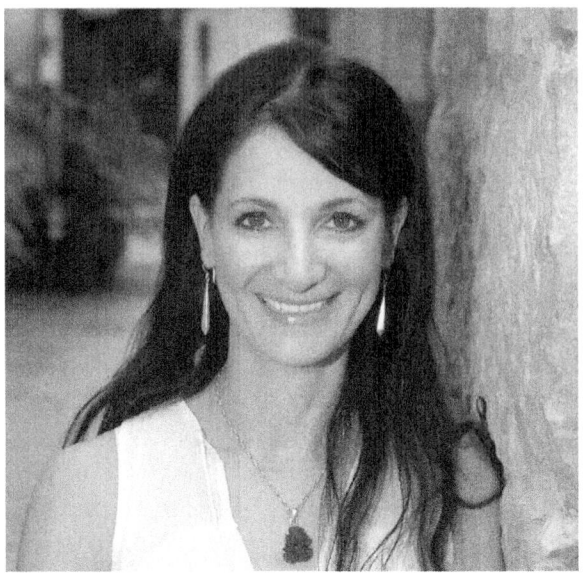

I'm a Mindfulness Coach and Well-being practitioner with a background in massage, energetic healing and Transformational Kinesiology. An illness redirected my life-path over twenty years ago which is when I immersed myself in learning about various healing arts. My interest in this field has continued to grow and I'm particularly fascinated by the mind, body and soul connection. I work in guiding people to reconnect with their inner being, which I believe is a source of love, truth and power. It is essential for our own personal wellbeing, as well as for that of the planet, that we become more conscious of the way we live our lives. There is great power that resides within each of us.

Now more than ever due to the fast pace lives we are living, I strongly believe that it is important for people to prioritise and care for their minds. The health of our mind is critical to the quality and overall wellbeing of our lives. Who doesn't want a life of joy, creativity, love, abundance and vitality!

Meditation is a very big part of my life. Having taught meditation workshops and witnessing the benefits of this ancient practice first hand, I was inspired to create a meditation app with my dear friend Eugenie Pepper. "Key Mindfulness" is created from a place of love, to promote peace of mind and nurturing wherever it may be needed. I firmly believe that the key to our wellbeing resides within each of us.

If you would like to learn more about us, please visit our website: www.keymindfulness.com

Or try one of our guided meditations: "The Key For Me" download the app Link: https://itunes.apple.com/au/app/key-for-me/id1318026274

YOUR WELL-BEING AND MIND AND BODY

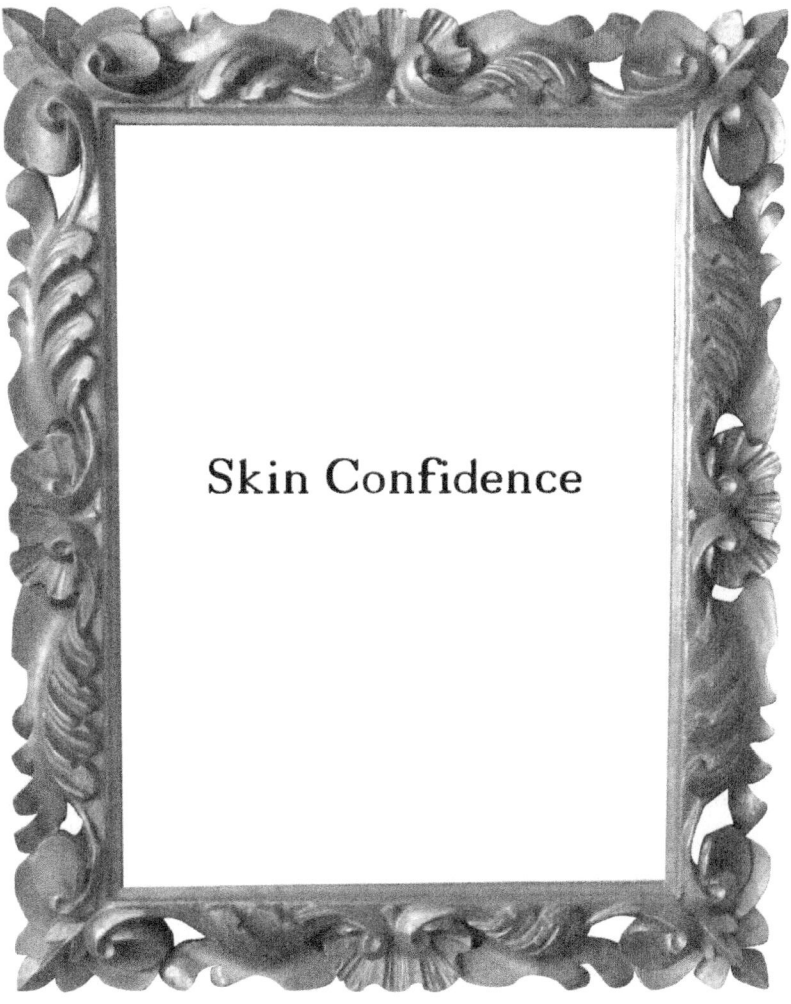

Skin Confidence

Skin Confidence

Our skin is our body's largest organ, which is pretty impressive. It protects our entire body and other organs, enables our movement, insulates (and waterproofs!) us and regulates our temperature. Our skin is our first defence against infection and its continual self-renewal and ability to heal and grow is remarkable. Brimming with nerves, our skin allows us to feel both pain and pleasure. It deserves respect from us from our head to our toes.

It's important that we look after our skin and learn how to work WITH it not AGAINST it – even if it gives us grief from time to time. Rather than rant and rave about our skin problems, we should take a step back and take time to learn what it likes and doesn't like. How it reacts to the products we use. The difference eating certain foods can make and how our quality of sleep, exercise and stress reduction contribute to not just how our skin looks, but how we feel towards it and, ultimately, ourselves.

When we speak about skin confidence, nine times out of 10 we are talking about the skin on our face as it is here where it – and we – are most exposed. Which is why our confidence can take a hit when we experience skin problems such as spots, breakouts or full-blown acne. My own personal experience, combined with working as a beautician for over 20 years, has helped me fully understand the impact of spots or acne is far more than simply skin deep.

When I was a teenager in the 1980s, I had what was referred to as 'bad skin'. No-one spoke to me about it which I thought was a blessed relief – I didn't want to discuss how hurt I felt. I hung my head, 'got on with it' and hoped I could get through each day without being teased or laughed at. The 'best' advice I was given was to squeeze the spots and put toothpaste on them overnight. Yes, seriously.

I remember writing to Cathy, the agony aunt at *Jackie* magazine, asking what I should do. Now it seems a crazy thing to have done, but at the time I felt it was my best chance. These days we speak more openly to our children: I'm already talking to my pre-teen sons about everything! But back then I didn't know what else to do. There was no internet to search, no social media to share my pain and no product reviews at my fingertips. There was also nowhere near the knowledge or appreciation that we have today of the benefits of natural products to nourish our skin. Neither was there awareness of the social and mental impacts of losing confidence in your looks to the point some people literally cannot face the world.

It's no wonder we struggle with acne, spots, breakouts and other troubling skin conditions: innately we are self-conscious if we have poor skin, especially on our face.

What has changed since my teenage years is the wealth of information we can now access, an appreciation of the impact having bad skin can have on someone's confidence and self-esteem and a more open society that allows us to talk more easily. We can find more information, search the latest reviews and listen to others in person or virtually to learn what has helped them. The fact you're reading this is proof we have moved on considerably: this greater knowledge and empathy are powerful!

Why me?

Good question – and one my teenage-self asked daily. Acne and oily skin can run in families it's true. But we can't blame our parents completely – skin problems are mainly triggered by a surge of hormones which leads to the over-production of the skin's oil-producing glands which form too much sebum.

This makes the skin and hair greasy and can block pores. The biggest hormonal changes that can cause acne, spots and breakouts occur during our teenage years, throughout our menstrual cycle, during pregnancy and the menopause. These factors we cannot control: but the additional triggers of breakouts – such as stress, unhealthy lifestyle choices and resorting to harsh chemicals and medication – can be moderated.

Spot: the difference

Spots are not created equal and there are different types that form including: blackheads, whiteheads, papules, pustules, nodules and cysts. They can vary in size, inflammation, pain and redness. Acne and spots can be sore due to what's going on <u>under</u> the skin: the temptation to pick or squeeze spots is strong but because of what's going on far deeper in your skin, it will have little effect and can create scarring. This is why you must leave your spots alone and NOT SQUEEZE. As mentioned before, our skin has an incredible potential to heal – let it do its job.

While it's clear that applying toothpaste won't help you much, using a specially created product to help calm and clear your skin makes perfect sense. But anyone who has started looking for solutions will be dazzled by the array of products and their claims. How do you know what's best to use?

Nature knows best

It makes sense to use natural products. We now understand far more the effects of what we eat and put 'in' our bodies but need to take the same care with what we feed our skin from the outside.

That sounds simple enough but beware as there are some nasty ingredients hidden in some products: even in those that sound and look gentle and 'natural'. You'd be right to assume that any over-the-counter or prescription products are medicated but some products on-the-shelf may also not be kind to your skin. Here are a few of the commonly used ingredients, treatments and medication that are best avoided.

Ingredients

Benzyl Peroxide can cause over-production of sebum as it strips the natural oils, can irritate the skin and make it more sensitive.

Alcohol can dry out the skin stripping away its much-needed natural oils and cause over-production of sebum.

SLS is also used as a car degreaser! It is so inflammatory, it's not allowed in non-wash off products.
Parabens, Phthalates, Triclosan have been shown to disrupt hormones.

Treatments

Laser or Light Therapy are for inflammatory acne and Laser Re-surfacing for post-acne scarring. They MUST be given by a qualified surgeon.
Extractor Pens are used to remove blackheads and whiteheads.
Chemical Peels are applied and the skin peeled off to reveal fresh, new (vulnerable) skin.

Prescribed Medications

Contraceptive Pill which can further disrupt hormones and sometimes make acne worse.
Antibiotics (eg: erythromycin, tetracycline and clindamycin) will attack both good and bad bacteria.
Retinoids (eg: tretinoin, isotretinoin and adapalene) can strip the skin of its natural oils and make it more sensitive and irritated.
Azelaic Acid can cause irritation and sensitivity.
Co-cyprindiol is a hormonal treatment.
Isotretinoin – Accutane – Roaccutane can cause many devastating side-effects including depression, suicide, harm to an unborn child and gut problems.

To prescribe or not?

It is worrying that prescribed medications are on the rise, especially for the last option above. It works for some but not for others. And even where it works to help the skin condition improve, the side-effects remain a huge concern: especially among teenagers and young adults who are highly susceptible to depression and suicide. As a beautician and skincare expert, I have spoken to many people who have taken prescription drugs to treat skin problems. Those whose skin has improved have experienced other problems, and over-dry skin.
For those where it hasn't worked, they have suffered with dry mouth and lips, discomfort in their gut and personal areas as well as depression and dark thoughts. With mental health, depression and suicide on the increase, it doesn't seem right to prescribe a drug to someone who is already depressed and unhappy which has a side-effect of depression and worse. This is my personal view but I can't help feeling medication is prescribed too readily before other options are explored. It should be an absolute LAST resort and then watched very carefully. These medications all have a list of side-effects. Bearing that in mind, it makes sense to try alternatives first. Patience is also needed here: everything will take time to take effect – even medication isn't a 'quick fix'.

If you're already on medication, you could look to move away from it and over to more natural products: getting used to a regular natural skincare routine whilst on medication is perfectly fine to do. I know several youngsters and older adults who have come off their medication – some after many years taking it – and found success using SkinGenius. A word of warning however: don't just stop the medication. You must consult your GP first as it may be important to lower the dose and come off it gradually.

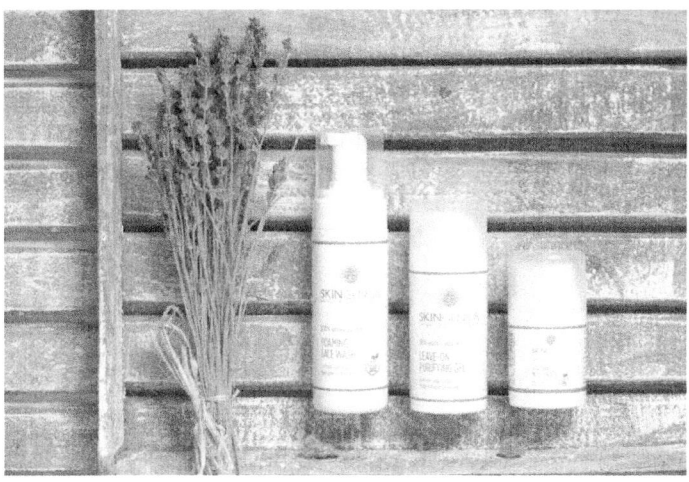

Ours are not the only natural products on the market – there is a wealth of choice now. I would urge anyone with skin problems to look at products that work with their skin to address the causes (and not just the symptoms) of acne, breakouts and pimples. Nourishing your skin and choosing natural over synthetic is the ultimate self-care.

It's time to redefine what we mean by 'treating' our skin. Consider the word 'treat' in its holistic, emotional, uplifting and rewarding sense, rather than its medical, fix-the-problem sense. Put another way, think positive and 'treat' your skin, and yourself, in more ways than one.

Start young for happy skin

If you have young children in your family, encourage them from around aged eight to get into a good routine. Prevention is better than cure! It's a great idea to get them into a routine of cleaning and cleansing BEFORE they experience any issues. Using a simple rose-water to start with is ideal and sticking with natural products will bring many more benefits than chemicals. From when my boys were born, I only ever used olive oil in their baths and on their skin and they never had eczema or other problems that affected some of their friends. On the few occasions they have tried off-the-shelf products, their skin dried out straight away: even pre-teen they can tell the difference.

Routine is key and you must stick to it: morning and night, seven days a week. Changes won't happen if you only use products for a few days or a couple of weeks. You must stay with it and give any new products at least three months to really see what they can do for you. A bit like changing your diet or trying a new fitness regime, skincare takes time to take effect: patience – and commitment – will bring results.

A good routine – cleanse, treat, moisturize

Cleansing your skin removes the day's dirt and bacteria that have been thrown at you. It will remove impurities, excess oil and clogged skin cells leaving your skin feeling fresh and clear.

Treating your clean skin with a treatment gel or lotion that sinks deeper into the layers of the skin will work to fight and prevent the bacteria that cause acne and spots. You will get the full benefits of doing this at night, as you have no other interferences and nature can peacefully work its magic while you sleep.

Moisturising with a light product that is non-comedogenic (won't block your pores) will bring lasting hydration, soothed skin cells, brightness and calm to your complexion.

Other tips

- Wash your hair regularly and keep it away from your face to help keep your skin clear.
- Avoid touching your face or affected areas as much as possible to minimise the transfer of infection, bacteria and dirt
- Use products wherever you have acne or breakouts – such as your back, neck, chest and arms
- Opt for gentle and natural make-up: mineral brands have fewer chemicals and oil in them so will be kinder to your skin.

Tried – and trusted

Some of the best therapies and botanical ingredients used today have been around for thousands of years, originating from remedies, yoga, homeopathy, reflexology and meditation. There's a reason why - natural ingredients work and can give fantastic results including a clear, calm and radiant skin.

It's important that we use and take advantage of the many wonderful ingredients we have at our fingertips which can bring a wealth of benefits to our skin. Natural ingredients are truly amazing: just one ingredient will have several properties within it to help different problems and reward you generously.

On the following page are a few of my favourite ingredients – I explain their benefits and why I love them so much. They are particularly good for people with acne, spots or blemishes. Look out for them in products: you can also buy them on their own to experiment with in your homemade recipes if you wish.

Witch Hazel (Hamamelis Virginiana)
It's at the top of my list! I have fond memories of Witch Hazel as a child: my grand-mother loved it and always had it in the garden and used it religiously every day. It is the go-to perfect natural cleanser for your skin and is a medicinal plant that has stood the test of time for hundreds of years. It helps reduce the growth of bacteria on the skin as well as preventing it producing excess oil. The tannins in this plant make it a natural astringent that can reduce and clear the pores while the high levels of healing active ingredients help speed up the clearing of infections. It also helps reduce signs of ageing, inflammation, cellular damage and swelling whilst soothing wounds and calming the skin. Witch Hazel is a natural antioxidant making it the perfect partner for your skin. It can be found in many products, but some will have other ingredients which may not be so kind to your skin so choose wisely. You can dilute it yourself with still or rose water or with an oil such as jojoba or rosehip and apply to the skin to give great results.

Calendula (Calendula Officinalis)

This is an absolute wonder herb to treat acne and spots. Its antimicrobial properties cleanse the skin from the main bacterium that causes acne (staphylococcus) and it soothes inflammation and reduces redness. The healing properties of Calendula have been proven to help speed the healing process of blemishes and acne scars.

Oregan Grape (Berberis Vulgaris)

This contains a compound called berbamine which kills on contact the bacteria that contribute to acne. It has significant antibacterial and anti-inflammatory properties that can help to heal your skin.

Nettle (Urtica Dioica)

Nettle is a master ingredient which is high in antioxidants that help to protect and heal the skin, reduce redness and ease swelling. It has anti-inflammatory, astringent and anti-bacterial qualities. Drinking nettle tea will bring health benefits too.

You can make your own by carefully picking the small shoots at the top of the plant to avoid being stung and brewing in boiling water for a few minutes. The nettle plant is considered to have numerous health benefits – including flushing toxins out of your body, lowering blood pressure, managing blood sugar levels and helping you cope with hay fever. So, not just an annoying rash-giving plant endured on country walks!!

Macadamia (Macadamia Ternifolia)

Its profile is similar to sebum, the oil which when produced in excessive quantities can lead to spots. Macadamia signals to the body to slow down sebum production helping to minimise this key cause of blocked pores. Macadamia is rich in anti-oxidants, gentle in action and has an anti-inflammatory action to help cool and soothe the skin. Macadamia nuts are a tasty treat too: they contain high levels of magnesium, which is also beneficial to healing your skin.

Yarrow (Achillea Millefolium)

Yarrow helps to control sebum production making it a 'must have' for anyone with acne, spots and oily skin. It is a natural astringent and a great skin healer which also helps to reduce scarring. It will calm and soothe the skin, reduce inflammation and redness and, being antimicrobial, can also fight the bacteria that cause acne and breakouts.

Hazelnut (Corylus Avellana)

Apart from being a great snack and full of goodness, hazelnuts help to control the body's own oil production. Packed with antioxidants plus Vitamins A and E, they help stimulate the regeneration of skin cells, leaving the skin feeling smooth and hydrated. It contains essential fatty acids that help moisturise the skin and boost its collagen to encourage elasticity.

Any of the above oils can be used at home mixed with a carrier oil such as jojoba, rose-hip or almond for a quick and easy fix for troubled skin.

More than skin deep

Acne and spots don't just affect our skin: they can strip away our confidence, enjoyment of social interaction and overall happiness. On bad days, bad skin can leave us wanting to stay under the duvet, avoid other people and even miss school, college or work. Having lived through it myself I know this is not an exaggeration: bad skin goes more than skin deep and it takes more than simply skin care to combat the behavioural, social and emotional impacts of acne, breakouts and unsightly spots.

Here are a few small changes that can make a big difference. You may be doing some of these already, in which case try and take them up to the next level and see how that feels.

Jot it down

There is little evidence to say that certain foods will cause acne but plenty to suggest that your skin and body will benefit from having a healthy diet. Listen to your gut and emotions and keep a diary of what you eat to track how certain foods and drinks make you feel physically and mentally. Writing it down will mean you don't overlook the 'occasional' food or drink that so many of us consume without even registering. (They could be the culprit so note everything down.) Make a note too on days you feel blue or brighter, if more spots appear or go, if you have more energy or not and what you did that day - work, study, go out with friends etc. You may see a pattern emerge and can then look at what is working for you and drop what's not.

More fruit and veg

You will see several changes in your body just by eating more fruit and veg. These help with your digestion, will make you more regular, give you longer lasting energy and a clearer outlook. Don't radically change your diet overnight, that's scary stuff and will probably go wrong. Maybe cut back on protein and carbohydrate sizes and add more veg to your plate, switch a mid-morning biscuit for a piece of fruit and add some berries to your morning cereal. Then start looking at new foods to ring the changes at mealtimes.

Drink up

What you drink and how often will have an effect on your skin and health. Drinking more water or herb teas each day will help to keep your head, skin and body clear. It's OK to enjoy coffee each day and a glass of wine a few evenings a week but be mindful of how much you're drinking and the timing. Limit caffeinated drinks to before midday to avoid disrupting your sleep later and have a few days each week without alcohol to allow your body to flush through the toxins.

Get out more!

Time outside in the fresh air and exercise will boost your mood. Even 15/20 minutes a day will make a difference. If you're at school or work all day, think about walking there (or partway) or back or take a walk at lunchtime. Go to the park with your friends after school, enjoy a family dog walk or simply saunter round the block with your partner before supper. Running, cycling, exercise classes, gym workouts and team sports are all excellent for your health and wellbeing and help flush toxins from your system. However, working up a sweat can irritate your acne so cleanse deeply and shower quickly after exercise to keep your skin as boosted as your spirits.

Get more shut-eye

Burning the candle at both ends isn't good for our stress levels, let alone our skin. Sleep is 'poor man's medicine' – a good eight hours a night will work wonders for your entire being. Going to bed earlier is better and easier to manage than sleeping in later, especially if you're at school, college or work. Sleep is not only precious for your mental state, your skin will love you for it too. Your body repairs itself while you're asleep and that includes regeneration of skin cells – inside and out.

A good night's sleep will reduce your levels of cortisol. Known as the 'stress hormone', it also triggers more sebum production which, in turn, can result in more spots. Blood flow increases at night and your skin produces more collagen which makes it more plump and can also reduce dark circles and puffy eyes.

- Try going to bed an hour earlier – start by going to bed 10 minutes earlier, then when you're used to that, 10 minutes earlier again and so on until your regular bedtime allows you at least seven or eight hours before the alarm goes off.
- Put down phones and ipads at least an hour before bed to help your mind switch off. Keep all 'flickering screens' out of the bedroom – invest in a good old-fashioned alarm clock and have that by your bedside.
- No distractions = better sleep.

Live YOUR life

Despite all the influences around us, we are ultimately responsible for how we live our lives. Choose to live yours well. Be mindful about how to make the most of each day. You may need to break some bad habits – as well as pick up some better ones! – but don't go making radical changes all at once. It takes around 12 weeks to fully break or make a habit. Introduce changes bit by bit and cut back rather than cut out. Gradually you will see and feel improvements and be spurred on to continue the better habit.

Silence your inner critic

We all let our inner critic, chimp or whatever you want to call it (mine's called Sid!) in at times and allow it to make us feel guilty about our behaviour, looks and decisions. A little of this keeps us questioning and registering our behaviour but too much becomes damaging to our psyche. Be confident to accept your inner criticism but find a way to deal with it when it gets too much. I talk, even shout, at Sid sometimes – it feels good to take back control, having registered the criticism I levelled at myself.

How others see you

Having suffered with acne as a teenager and young adult I know first-hand how it feels. The social isolation, shying away from people and feeling supremely self-consciousness even with my closest friends and family.

I remember a photo being taken when I was about 15 that revealed my face full of spots topped off with a big 80s perm! That photo is long gone – I threw it away with so many others that I had hated being taken. Nowadays with selfies, Snapchat stories and Insta, the trauma of being captured in photos that are instantly circulated is acute. Try and remember, though, whether in a photo or in person, people don't see what you see. Yes, they can see your spots, breakout or redness but they are not critical or loathing of them as you may be. They see you – and beyond your problem skin.

Love the skin you're in

Attitudes in society and tolerance have moved on massively since my teenage years – alternative looks, be they natural or created, are accepted more readily and the recent movement to love the skin you're in and embrace people and ourselves as we are naturally is empowering. That's not to say if you have problem skin you shouldn't do all you can to clear it. You will look and feel better for it.

But, while you're working on clearing your skin and living through hormonal upsets and such like, don't put your social life and friendships on hold. Instead, embrace them, live your life, get out more and enjoy yourself. In doing so, your confidence will grow and you will have less time to dwell on your skin condition and it will no longer define you.

Keep calm and carry on

Be patient, find what works for you and remember there is no such thing as an overnight success when it comes to skin improvements. Be accepting of yourself and your skin: take steps to improve your skincare routine, introduce natural products, eat healthy foods, have more sleep and take daily exercise. Each day will become a little bit easier. As I sit here writing I have some spots on my face and the back of my neck: thanks to me approaching the menopause. But it's different this time round as I know how to treat my skin and adhere to my skincare routine with natural products, enjoy a better diet and a healthier outlook.

I've made positive choices to opt for natural and organic products that work with my skin and to live a lifestyle that suits me well. I am sharing this with my friends and family as well as with you. It's not a taboo – it's life!

Be kind to yourself

Be kind to yourself; treat yourself to the best skincare, diet and lifestyle choices you can manage and hold your head high. Keep it real – you're not an airbrushed image; you're a living, breathing being with heart, soul, energy, love and warmth to bring to the day. Confidence comes from within: from knowing you're doing your best to be your best. Smile and step lightly. At SkinGenius our message is *'Be Clear, Be Confident, Be You.'* It's a positive mantra that I try to live by. I hope it helps you too.

By Julia Vearncombe

About the author

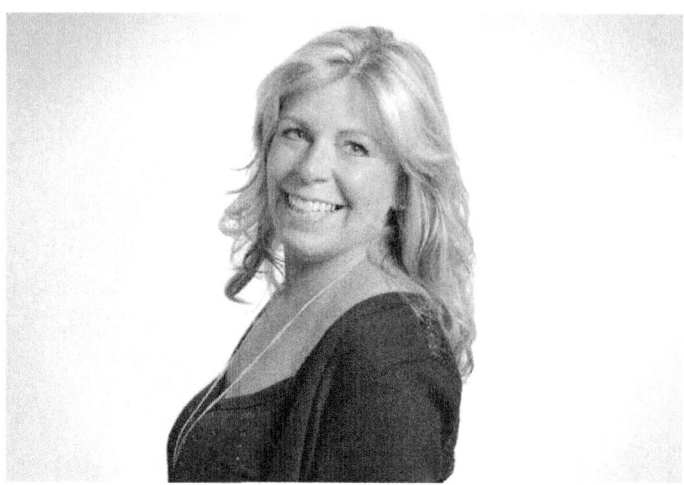

I am 48 and a beautician and hairdresser by trade. In recent years I have met many clients who had skincare problems and/or were parents of teens and pre-teens who are struggling to find effective solutions that are natural and would work effectively.

I did a lot of research to find suitable solutions but could find none. There was a definite gap in the market for natural skincare for people struggling to combat acne and troublesome skin.

I was also seeing too many people in my salon and at the school gates who were on medication for skin conditions, struggling daily with oily skin, breakouts, flushed complexions and the anxiety that goes with it all. I partnered with homeopath Hilery Dorrian to create SkinGenius.

I'm passionate about the power of natural ingredients to restore harmony not only to the skin but also to our happiness and wellbeing. I have worked closely with homeopaths and natural skincare specialists to develop an accessible, affordable range. The positive results we have seen has restored people's skin confidence and I'm delighted to say it's not unusual for people to tell me our products have 'changed their life'. It's not always easy defying convention – me in creating these products and my customers in trying them. But when they work so well and people show me their skin has cleared I know, 100%, that I'm doing the right thing.

www.skin-genius.co.uk

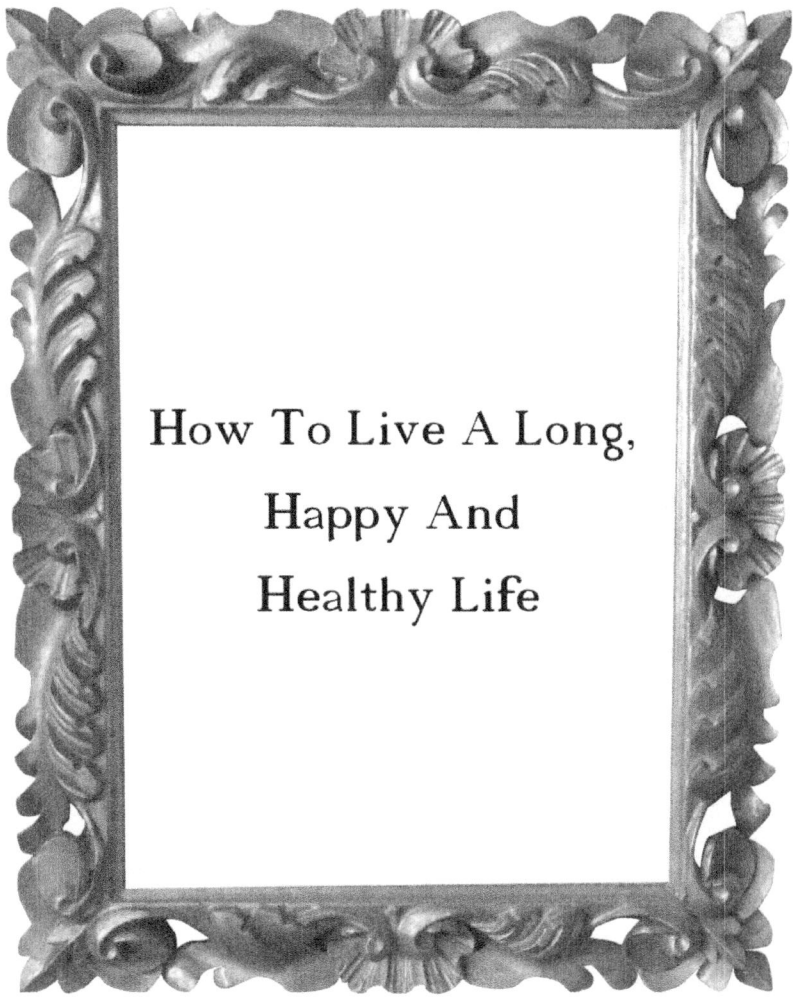

How To Live A Long, Happy And Healthy Life

How To Live A Long, Happy And Healthy Life

Who doesn't want to age well? Who doesn't want to minimise the length of time they experience poor health before departing this world? Death is inevitable but an extended period of poor health is not. Ageing well isn't just about how long we live but about how long we feel vital and happy and about how long we can keep doing the things we enjoy. Much of the chronic disease associated with old age is lifestyle related. I am fascinated by the science behind longevity and here, in this chapter, I have tried to bring together some of the most useful and beneficial tips and healthy lifestyle habits which you can start to incorporate into your life today. I have assembled the tips under 8 pillars of health – Mindset, Food and Drink, Movement, Breathing, Sleep, Self-Care, Life Purpose and Our Environment.

Our MINDSET is very important when it comes to healthy ageing. A positive or growth mindset has a positive impact on our health. Research has shown that the mind is so powerful that it can influence health outcomes. So, evaluating our thoughts is key to assessing whether we have a growth mindset or fixed mindset.

A fixed mindset means we don't have an open mind - that we see ourselves as unchanging. A fixed mindset means we are probably afraid of change and afraid of making mistakes, and that we feel change isn't worth the effort. Someone with a fixed mindset tends to be self-critical and this, in itself, can prevent them from making change. Negativity puts stress on the body and long-term stress and high levels of cortisol, the stress hormone, can impact heart health, sleep, weight and cognitive health.

A growth mindset embraces change. Someone with a growth mindset is looking for ways to improve (their health or their business etc.) and while change is hard, those with a growth mindset recognise the potential benefits of change. These people tend to be mentally resilient, have better relationships, better focus, less stress and anxiety. It is likely that someone with a growth mindset has a positive attitude towards ageing. The better our attitude towards ageing, the better our experience of ageing is likely to be.

Some people seem to be blessed with a growth mindset but it is probably a personality trait learnt in childhood. Even if we have a fixed mindset we can change – we all have the ability to become more growth minded. Reframing negative thoughts can be useful. If you are struggling with something – at work or at home – try to see it as a challenge rather than a problem and as an opportunity to rise to the occasion. We can also reframe negative thoughts about our lives and about ourselves. For example, rather than getting up in the morning and saying how dreadful the weather is or how awful you look, try to reframe your thoughts – so you might think or say instead how much the garden needs the rain or how good you will feel after a walk or a shower etc. Starting your day with a positive mindset sets you up for a good day. So, pay attention to your thoughts and speak to yourself as you would speak to a friend. Some self-compassion and expressing gratitude for small things helps bring about a positive mindset. If you take a walk view your surroundings and try to lookout for positive things like flowers in a garden or a cute dog! Always look on the bright side of life ... Our mindset can also be improved by focusing on the journey rather than the destination. This is particularly true of our health – our health is a journey. We often spend too much time focused on thoughts like "I'll be happy when I have lost 10kg" or I need to be fit before I do park run etc. Focus on the journey and enjoy it! Optimists generally have better health than pessimists – this doesn't mean you have to put on a fake front of jollity but by believing in yourself, reframing negative thoughts, listening to your body, and speaking kindly to yourself you will put yourself in a good place and improve your chances of healthy longevity.

HOW, WHAT, WHERE AND WHEN WE EAT AND DRINK

I couldn't write a chapter on healthy ageing without talking about food and drink!!

Let's start by considering what we eat and drink. It is generally accepted that a Mediterranean style diet promotes healthy longevity. A Mediterranean style diet is full of vegetables, fruit, nuts, seeds, legumes, whole grains, some fish and a little dairy and meat if you choose. Make vegetables the stars of your plate! Where possible we should be eating food that is fresh, natural and real. We want to avoid ultra-processed foods – this isn't just fast food or junk food. This is food that is packaged with scary sounding ingredients and an equally scary shelf or fridge life. Tim Spector, in his brilliant book Spoon-Fed, tells us to beware of mis-leading food labelling. Certain ultra-processed foods may be labelled as "healthy", "natural", "organic" or "low fat" and while these words may describe some of the original ingredients, they don't refer to the process of how the food was made and the final outcome. Tim Spector also says that we need to be aware that not all processed food is bad – frozen vegetables are processed as is a good quality artisanal loaf of sourdough bread. What is important is that we understand the difference between that loaf of bread and the slimy white sliced version sitting on the supermarket shelf.

If you can, eat organic. Pesticides mess with our immune systems. Try to eat a wide variety of different vegetables and other phytonutrients (things that grow in the ground!) – aim for 30 different phytonutrients a week. It is not as hard as it sounds if you make use of herbs and spices, nuts and seeds as well as vegetables, fruit and whole grains. Build up your repertoire slowly, introducing a couple of new ingredients every week. Using a weekly colour chart on your kitchen wall can be motivating and fun to do with children.

Cooking from scratch can seem time consuming but try to carve out some time for meal preparation. Make it part of your weekly schedule. Just by planning your meals and your shopping can make eating like this simpler. If it all feels completely new to you, start by tackling certain aspects of your diet. Don't get caught up with particular "diets" like paleo or keto. They may have a role to play in certain medical situations but, generally speaking, most people will benefit from favouring a Mediterranean style of diet. Learn to listen to your body and work out how you respond to different foods. We are all unique so just because your friend follows a vegan diet and raves about the health benefits, it may not be right for you.

We all know that drinking water is important for our health and I am sure we have all experienced the knock-on effects of dehydration such as headaches and constipation. Filtered tap water is fine and, in many ways, preferable to bottled water. We read mixed messages about alcohol. Drinking heavily is clearly detrimental to our health -it leads to alcoholism, liver disease and mental health problems. Some observational studies indicate that one or two drinks a day is ok but other studies indicate that any alcohol, particularly for women, is detrimental to health. What we do know is that people break down alcohol differently. If you metabolise alcohol quickly so less gets into the bloodstream, there will be fewer effects on the body and you will become less intoxicated than someone else. Women in menopause seem less able to metabolize alcohol and their resistance goes down. Moderate alcohol consumption can bring pleasure and can be social both of which are important for longevity and mental health. I really enjoy a glass of wine or two with a good meal eaten with family or friends. I guess it's all about moderation!

Coffee can also get a bad rap in the press. Again, we all have different responses to caffeine and it is worth spending some time assessing how coffee affects you. I prefer not to drink coffee after about 1pm as it impacts my sleep. It is thought that coffee in the afternoon may well impact the quality of your sleep whether or not you are aware of any sleep disturbance so think about that next time you drink coffee in the evening. Coffee contains polyphenols, the plant chemicals found in much fruit and veg, and fibre which is fermented in our colon to produce short chain fatty acids which help the beneficial bacteria in our guts flourish! As with anything we consume, aim to drink the best quality coffee you can.

So now onto where, how, and when we eat and drink. When possible eat your meals at a table. Our posture when eating impacts our digestion. Avoid eating on the move, in your car or slumped on the sofa. Try to eat mindfully so put down your phone and focus on your meal, the colours and the textures etc Eat slowly and chew your food properly. The digestive process starts when you see or smell your food and chewing/breaking down your food is also a big part of this process. I ask my clients to tune into their hunger and fullness signals too. This can take time and practice but it helps to eat when we are just hungry not starving and to finish eating when we are 75% full, not stuffed. This obviously helps with weight management, but also with our food choices, our digestion and our energy levels.

Time restricted eating or intermittent fasting is very fashionable at the moment but it isn't new and it isn't a fad. Short fasts can benefit us in a few ways. One is a simple calorie reduction. Frank Lipman, author of The New Rules of Ageing Well, says that the biggest factor in healthy ageing is eating less. Over the age of 45, we don't need as many calories. He certainly isn't advocating calorie counting and of course it rather depends on how much you are currently eating. Consuming less food gives our body a break – our digestive system works better if it has a chance to rest and recover. Fasting also impacts crucial hormones that affect ageing and weight including insulin and growth hormone. Fasting is also a small stressor, like a cold shower, that stimulates our longevity gene pathways. Fasting also kick starts autophagy, the cellular detox process, critical to strong immunity and ageing well. Frank Lipman recommends a 16 hour overnight fast but others recommend at least 12 hours. Jeanette Hyde, nutritionist, after much research and working with women in her clinic, recommends that women fast over night for 14 hours. She says that focusing on eating earlier in the day is best but for many an early evening meal isn't always practical. Try it and find what works for you. Again for many of us, it is hard to do. I always suggest trying it on one or two days a week. It depends where you are starting from. If you're a late night snacker maybe work on cutting this out first of all. Try to identify why you snack – is it because you are hungry or is it an emotional response?

My next set of tips revolve around **MOVEMENT**. I am a Personal Trainer as well as a Health Coach so I am afraid all my clients get the strength training lecture! Maintaining muscle mass is critical as we get older. Sarcopenia or muscle loss kicks in from the age of around 30 and after the age of 40 we lose about 1% of our muscle mass per year. Unfortunately for women in peri menopause it is likely that this figure is closer to 3%. At around the age of 60/65 we need to increase our protein intake as well as working on our strength. Strength training isn't just about lifting weights – it is any activity which involves resistance so we can use our body weight – think squats, lunges, planks and push ups or we can use stretchy bands, dumbbells and kettle bells. Keep some dumbbells in the kitchen and do a few arm exercises while you wait for the kettle to boil! Building muscle is not just about us staying strong and flexible. Muscle is linked to improved cell function, reduced inflammation, better cognition and slower bone loss. This is particularly important for women in midlife and older who don't take HRT (hormone replacement therapy) as they are at greater risk of developing osteoporosis.

Cardio workouts are also important as is balance work. Cardio exercise boosts blood flow, multiplies mitochondria(the energy powerhouses in our cells), brings more oxygen to our muscles, builds endurance and switches on longevity genes. You don't need to be running marathons though. Running is ok but be careful not to injure yourself. Walking with purpose so you get your heart rate up, swimming and cycling are good and possibly less likely to lead to injury than running.

Balance work is important too. Think about the main reasons older people fall. Strong core muscles and balance work help reduce falls. Try standing on one leg while brushing your teeth every morning. Add in some balance work to your strength training. For example, single leg squats, certain yoga poses such as the tree, single leg deadlifts, standing on a wobble cushion or Bosu for arm work etc

Plan your movement into your week. Make sure your routine is varied as it's good to mix up strength work with cardio and it also prevents you getting bored from doing the same routine week in and week out. Try a new activity such as paddle boarding or take up a dance class. Dancing requires a unique blend of strength, balance, endurance, memory and concentration so its great for our bodies and our brains! Researchers in Japan found that dancing is the best exercise to reduce the risk of functional decline i.e. being unable to look after ourselves.

Movement doesn't always have to mean prescribed exercise. Non-exercise activity thermogenesis (NEAT) is the energy expended for everything we do that is not sleeping, eating or sport-like exercise. So, this might include walking rather than going by car, cleaning your house, doing some gardening, even fidgeting. I am always telling my clients to get up from their desks at least every hour and walk around the house or do some stretching. In "blue zones" – those places around the world where people live exceptionally long, healthy lives, one of the common features across all regions is daily movement and lots of it. Make movement part of your lifestyle not just something you do twice a week at the gym.

My fourth pillar of health focuses on **BREATHING**. Breathwork is all the rage at the moment but there really is something in it. Breathwork is free and it helps you manage stress and anxiety, sleep better and release tension. I listened to Dr Andrew Weil, a pioneer in the field of integrative health, on a podcast recently. He has done a lot of research in the area of chronic inflammation now a widely accepted cause of many serious health conditions. In the podcast he talked about the importance of minimizing stress and how breathwork is a real game changer when it comes to managing stress. Stress is a clear example of the mind-body connection. Unmanaged chronic stress makes us ill and is profoundly ageing. Breathwork such as a simple 4-7-8 breathing pattern can have astounding benefits. Calm, centred breathing triggers the parasympathetic nervous system – our rest and digest system – sending positive messages to the brain which turns off the sympathetic/fight of flight nervous system. Breathe in through your nose for a count of 4, hold for 7 and breathe out for a count of 8. Do it for a few minutes. Sit or lie down and relax; draw the air down so that your belly expands; hold; then breathe out in a controlled fashion.

In his book The Oxygen Advantage, Patrick McKeown, explains how most of us over breathe and rather like overeating, it isn't good for our health or our longevity. Overbreathing means breathing more air than your body requires during rest and exercise. Overbreathing causes narrowing of the airways, limiting the body's ability to oxygenate, and the constriction of blood vessels, leading to reduced blood flow to the heart and other organs and muscles. We learnt at school that we breathe in oxygen and breathe out carbon dioxide. This is correct but what we didn't learn is that carbon dioxide is the key variable that allows the release of oxygen from our red blood cells to be metabolised by the body. The amount of carbon dioxide in our blood cells determines how much oxygen we can use and how we breathe determines carbon dioxde levels in our blood. If we are overbreathing we are exhaling too much carbon dioxide. People who overbreathe tend to breathe through their mouths so we need to switch to nasal breathing. This concept isn't new – yogis have been practicing nasal breathing for years. My advice to clients and something I myself practice is to nasal breathe at all times including when sleeping and exercising. If I feel out of breath when exercising I drop the intensity so that normal nasal breathing resumes. If you are a snorer, try taping your mouth at night. People record improved sleep duration and quality after doing this. And we all know how important sleep is for healthy ageing.

My fifth pillar of health is **SLEEP**. I could probably write a book on sleep there is so much to say. I have struggled with sleep for much of my adult life and the knowledge that it was impacting both my current and future health didn't really help!

If we want to live healthy, long lives then we need to prioritize our sleep. There are certain things we can do to support good sleep which I will briefly discuss below but it is worth saying at the outset that if poor sleep persists, seek help. I eventually sought help from a sleep specialist and that, together with having a full genome report done by Lifecode GX which helped me identify that taking a Melatonin supplement would support better sleep, has really helped. We are all individuals with our own unique DNA so what works for one person may not work for another. This is one reason why conventional medicine doesn't always work. As a Health Coach I encourage my clients to tune into their body and listen to the messages it is sending; to try different things and to work out what works best for them.

So here are a few tips that many people find helpful when it comes to getting a good night's sleep.
- Try to stick to a routine, so go to bed and rise in the morning at the same time every day; dim the lights in the evening and put away technology at least an hour before bed. Avoid watching the news before bed!
- Exercise every day and preferably in the morning.
- Get outside - morning sunlight helps keep our circadian rhythms in tune with nature.
- Make your bedroom a calming place to relax in so don't have technology, a TV or bright lights in there. Keep it dark and quiet. I wear an eye mask and often wear ear plugs.
- Many people find meditation and breathing exercises help. I certainly find breathing exercises help me when I wake at night. I focus on my breathing, slowing it down and then when I feel settled I either call to mind the colour blue or a calming place.
- Avoid eating late and cut back on alcohol and caffeine in the evening. Work out if you are sensitive to caffeine. How we metabolize caffeine is genetic so some people can drink it in the evening with zero effect (my husband!) and others can't drink it after midday (that's me!). Alcohol disrupts the sleep cycle plus wine and beer are high in carbs and turn to sugar in the body which in itself can affect sleep.
- Brain dump before you go to bed. Write down your "to do" list or anything that is bothering you. It really helps! And while you are at it, write down three things that have made you smile or feel happy that day.

Pillar number six is **SELF-CARE**. Self- care means different things to different people. It may mean treating yourself to a spa day, having a day out with friends, setting aside some me time to read a book, take a bath etc. It may also mean doing something about the Pillars of Health we have already looked at, taking some action to finally do the exercise, change your diet , start meditating and so on. Self-care is essential at every stage of life but many of us aren't very good at it. Our own health is often at the bottom of the "to do" list. Women in midlife typically juggle family life, teenage children or children leaving home, ageing parents, demanding careers and relationships problems. This can leave very little me time. There is truth in the saying that we can't pour from an empty cup. So schedule self-care into your week and prioritize this time.

Another aspect of self-care which is very important for healthy longevity is listening to your body – do not ignore aches and pains. If you are exercising, which I hope you are, stretch out those muscles and invest in a foam roller and roll out any tightness. Often it isn't muscle that is tight, it's fascia. Fascia is the stuff that encases our muscles and as we get older, it gets tighter! So, use a foam roller regularly – ask a Personal Trainer to show you how to use one. If foam rolling doesn't sort the problem then go and see a professional who can help. Do not let problems linger or they will most likely get worse not better. Make sure you are eating lots of magnesium rich foods too – dark green leafy veg, pumpkin seeds, whole grains, beans and dark chocolate because magnesium, amongst other things, helps with muscle relaxation, cramp etc You could also try taking an Epsom salts bath. Sauna sessions are also useful for achy muscles , pain due to inflammation and detoxification.

Your feet are essential when it comes to healthy longevity. Look after them. Go barefoot at home as much as possible; don't wear shoes that cause pain; switch your shoes around or wear barefoot shoes for day to day activities; and roll your feet out with a tennis ball or similar.

And ladies, look after your pelvic floors. So many older women are admitted to nursing homes because they are incontinent. If you are experiencing pelvic discomfort, leakage or worse then seek help. As oestrogen levels drop during peri menopause most women experience a change in the way in which their pelvic floor functions – it is not unusual to experience leakage but it doesn't have to be that way. Speak up, talk to your doctor or see a physiotherapist who specializes in pelvic floor health. A weak pelvic floor can be very distressing and can lead to mental health problems.

Finally, get your moles checked out. Don't ignore changes.

Pillar 7 is **LIFE PURPOSE**. Maintaining our interest in life and curiosity about the world around us is key to a happy, healthy life. Cultivating joy, calm, relationships and awareness are important aspects of ageing well. Loneliness is a marker for poor health so it is important that we work on social connection while it is relatively easy. Lifelong learning is also useful for our long-term brain health – it is never too late to learn a new skill and to challenge the brain. So read books which make you think, learn a language or learn to play a musical instrument – now that would be a real challenge for me! Doing something creative builds cognitive flexibility. Artistic creatives often don't retire in the traditional sense because what motivated them to work in the first place continues to motivate them as they get older. Such people often have a strong sense of life purpose and have an open and optimistic attitude towards life. Cognitive flexibility refers to an openness to new ideas and a flexible attitude towards change. Of course, non-artistic creatives can aspire to this kind of positive attitude and if they succeed it will serve them well in the healthy longevity stakes.

Blue Zones are regions of the world where a higher than usual number of people live longer than average. According to Blue Zone researchers, knowing your sense of purpose or why you wake up every morning is worth up to seven years of extra life expectancy and is linked to a reduced risk of Alzheimer's, stroke and arthritis. Take a step back and have a think about your reasons for wanting to age well. It may not be anything remotely unusual – quite possibly it will be something mundane like I want to see my grandchildren grow up and I don't want to be a burden. This is your WHY. And keep your WHY in mind when trying to implement any lifestyle habit changes that you want to implement after reading this chapter! Write your WHY down somewhere where you will see it every morning. My WHY is to avoid getting dementia and ending up in a care home like my mother; to be able to enjoy the company of my children and that of any grandchildren I am lucky enough to have; to play tennis until they kick me out of the tennis club and to keep spreading the message about how we can age healthily.

Finally Pillar 8: **OUR ENVIRONMENT** and while I am in favour of green government policies and action on climate change, this is more about our own environment. Think about what you put on your skin as well as what you put inside your body; think about the quality of the air in your home (unfortunately you can't do much about the air quality outside your home unless you move house!); and think about the utensils you use for cooking. What skin and make up products do you use? Your skin is an organ and what you put on it seeps into your bloodstream and becomes part of your microbiome. So, choose carefully when it comes to soap, shampoo, face products, deodorant, make up and perfume. Please don't use aggressive mouth washes – your mouth has its own microbiome and mouth washes can cause an imbalance which can in turn impact your immune health. You want to avoid chemicals. I suggest you use organic products and the market for this is taking off.
Likewise with cleaning products and air fresheners – most commercial versions of these are pretty toxic. Try using essential oils and diffusers instead of commercial sprays and candles. Research shows that keeping house plants improve air quality at home. Homemade cleaning products based on vinegar, essential oils and/bicarbonate of soda work well.

Think about what you cook with and how your food is wrapped. Use glass instead of plastic particularly in a microwave and wax wraps instead of cling film for covering food. When it comes to cooking utensils stainless steel, silicone or wood is best. Avoid Teflon/nonstick coated pans if you can. And when you are out and about avoid walking besides busy roads and take the side streets instead. By doing this you will be breathing in significantly less pollution.

My final message is this – embrace life, do what you enjoy and remember it is never too late to make lifestyle changes!

By Amanda Price

About the author

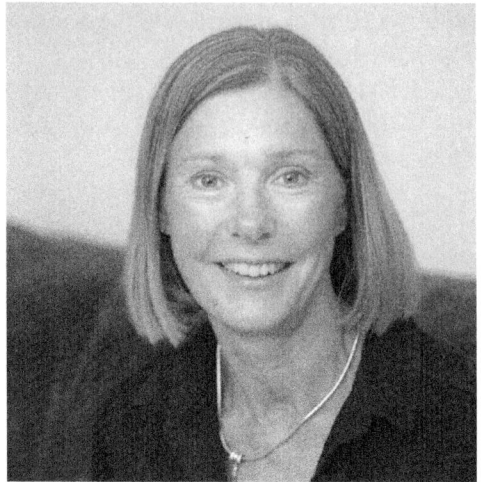

Amanda is a Women's Health Coach and Personal Trainer. She is a member of the UK Health Coach Association. She works both in person and online with women in midlife and older helping them to feel happier and healthier. She takes a whole- body view of health and is a diet agnostic. She uses a variety of techniques to promote lifestyle habit changes. She helps her clients manage their menopause symptoms, lose weight, gain physical and mental energy, better manage stress and reduce their risk of developing a chronic lifestyle disease such as heart disease, osteoporosis, dementia or type 2 diabetes. Amanda is passionate about helping women age healthily and happily. She works in partnership with her clients providing support, encouragement and accountability. You can contact her to arrange a free discovery chat which gives you the opportunity to find out how Amanda might be able to help you.

www.amandapricekirby.com
apkhealthandfitness@gmail.com
https://facebook.com/apkhealthandfitness
https://www.instagram.com/theagewellcoach
https://www.linkedin.com/in/amandapricekirby/

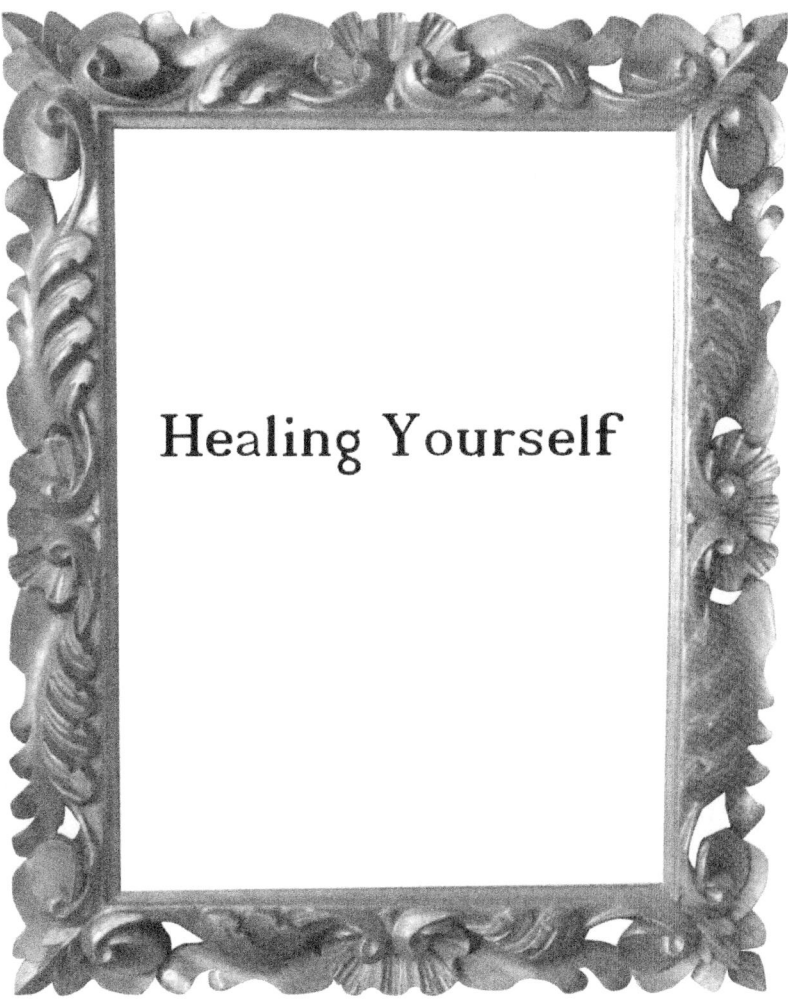

Healing Yourself

Healing Yourself

There is tremendous power in discovering how to help yourself. To come out of the fear and move into *here*. What is it to live a life defined by illness and diagnosis, the labelling by others of what is 'wrong' with you? This can translate to a person becoming their illness. It perfuses the very being of a human body and mind and informs the reality.

Whilst the 'what' of a diagnosis is interesting in terms of practical information, the far more delving questions beyond the superficiality of a clinical diagnosis, is why and how? So we then move into a position of empowerment where we can take action based on the information in hand rather than be consumed by it. We can ask of ourselves, ok what's really going on here. What is my body relaying to me? How can I best respond?

We can then grow and evolve from our experiences rather than be destroyed by them.

That is empowerment.

If you believe, as I do, that thoughts influence the body and more specifically the organisation of cells and tissue, this is an incredible connection to make for yourself as we then understand how our beliefs and unconscious patterns impact upon our health and wellbeing. Being well.

In turn it then makes complete sense that mastery over your mind is a key tool to your vitality. So you are not then just a body at the mercy of your thoughts or indeed the thoughts of others, you are a cohesive unit of undulating information that has the capacity to change in an instant.

This is a process that is unique to each person. Mastery of the mind is not about denying your feelings. It is important to be vigilant in honouring your emotions so they are truly felt and can then be released. So you are aware of them, you are bearing witness to them, and then able to let them go rather than choosing avoidance. Avoiding how you feel is where old patterns then have the power to sit behind you driving your future.

I developed kidney issues when a very young child. At the age of four, I contracted a strep throat, a bacterial infection that unusually localised to my kidneys precipitating a form of nephritis, inflammation in the tiny magnificent filters of the kidneys. Although a very healthy child in spite of this and under the care of a wonderful doctor in Johannesburg who had a very holistic approach, by the age of ten, having being sent away to boarding school in Dublin, I became ill due to the kidney issue. Far from the comfort of our Zambian home and the love of my parents, I was hospitalised. Reflecting back I now more fully appreciate the value of having the holistic care between the ages of four to ten.

I was on no medication, there was clear guidance from my doctor in South Africa to manage my health through food with limited refined sugar, plenty of water, wholesome food and no more vaccinations as with kidneys under duress, vaccinations can add to the burden. His advice took into account that I was a young child that needed to flourish. It was not a linear approach and certainly was in keeping with naturopathic principles, especially First Do No Harm. He was based in a hospital and was a paediatric nephrologist so the medical credentials were there but he had that wider understanding. He was also just a lovely kind man.

I know now that this early introduction to what truthful healthcare looks and feels like has informed my journey hugely. I felt safe and understood and not at all mistrustful of this doctor. This care, together with the gift of growing up in abundant Zambia where we had banana, papaya and avocado trees in our garden as well as a vegetable garden tended to by our lovely gardener Simeon, has informed me on how important our environment is to our wellbeing. I am blessed to have grown up in in this way.

I know this created in me an approach towards the understanding that there is so much we can do to keep ourselves well whilst navigating an ongoing illness, in whatever context that might manifest in your body. It can become your greatest opportunity to evolve and to experience what it is to have true perspective and to know yourself.

By age fourteen, my kidneys had reached a point where their function could no longer keep me well. My family by this time had relocated from beautiful Zambia to Dorset in the UK. I was now under the care of the UK health system which was a million miles away from the care I had in South Africa.

A highly medicalised and distant approach that was not in any way holistic or progressive. It was a bleak time in many respects but certainly not without hope. In spite of the bleakness, I would always return to an inner sense of hopefulness.

From age fourteen to twenty one I had haemodialysis to sustain me. Thrice weekly treatments where my blood would be filtered over a number of hours through an artificial kidney. This was something that I adapted to and just became part of my routine. That's not to say it was easy, there were many tough and harrowing experiences along the way but I remained a resilient teenager eager to live a full life with an inner knowing that I could always do something to help myself. I excelled at school, played on the tennis team, was appointed deputy head girl and achieved excellent GCSE grades going onto study A-levels and then university. At twenty one I received the call from hospital that there was a donor kidney for me. So off I went and had the gift of a kidney grafted into my left iliac crest, native kidneys left in situ.

A year after this surgery, I went travelling around the world with a good friend, twenty two by now, I was developing a stronger interest in wellbeing and felt very connected to the healing power of nature. Travelling in the heat of Australia reminded me of my beloved Zambia and childhood freedom. I felt the warmth of the sun through to my very bones.

I fell into a career in banking on returning home after our exciting world travels and settled in London. I met a man who I embarked on a deep relationship with, fell in love and we set up home together. Really I was living the expected life of a young adult; great job, great earning prospects, coupled up and engaged to be married. The end...

After five years this relationship finally buckled. Nursing a broken heart I started to slowly realise how I had not really felt my emotions and had disconnected from my heart and almost allowed this huge sadness to completely consume me. As such it took the next few years to unpick my childhood experience of renal failure, dialysis, transplantation and the intense drug regime of immuno-suppressants. It was at this time I re-discovered yoga, now in my late twenties. My best friend was raving about a class at the gym where we were working and encouraged me to go. I had had some exposure to yoga through my mom who trained in South Africa in the 70s for her certification and she would hold children's classes at our home in Zambia. Seemingly it was in my DNA.

Reconnecting with it as a woman in my late twenties by then was profound. I started to experience my body much more and take a greater interest in keeping it well. I played my guitar a lot more and sang, things that had been sadly neglected whilst in my previous relationship. I travelled widely and embraced the wonder that going to far flung places brings, how this is medicine for the soul. In my early thirties I started to feel a draw from within to explore health in a much deeper way and as synchronicity would have it, I happened upon a naturopathic nutrition course that just sounded perfect for me. As my best friend said at the time when I told her, 'Wow, that will fit you like a glove.'

The universe affirms good choices so you just know them to be right for you. My mom was also beyond thrilled when I told her. And so I enrolled for the three year course which meant most weekends for the following three years would be spoken for as I was attending college alongside my full-time city banking job. Rather than this feeling too much or overwhelming, it nurtured me and woke me up to a much more resonant world for me. I loved the course. I loved learning more about the intricacy of our human anatomy and its innate intelligence. I had the advantage of years of my own health experiences and so medical language was like second nature to me, especially when it came to kidneys. I had imbibed and absorbed a lot from the years of regular hospital exposure and understanding my own body. It was an incredibly comprehensive course and I felt ready to begin to see patients as soon as I qualified.

I had continued with a regular yoga practice during these years of study and had planted a seed of intention on a beach in the Perhentian Islands saying to my travelling companion, 'I'm going to do my yoga teacher training.' Vocalising an intention and having it witnessed can be very potent. It sends the ripples of intention outwards to be manifested. And so more and more I started to feel a bigger vision for myself, for my life of service to others and deeply trusting my instincts.

I decided to resign from my job and amazingly the global head of credit risk at the time offered me to go part time. Another massive sign of support. The role I did was not typically suited to part time but it all worked out. I went off to complete a month-long yoga immersion in Spain to learn to teach this wonderful wisdom and returned home to London sliding into a three day working week. This allowed me time to focus on building my own business whilst still having a healthy income and so my wellbeing business Wholly Aligned was borne.

Along came a big awakening in 2013. Only three or four months into the part time hours and now a qualified yoga teacher, I began to feel unwell. It seemed my transplant kidney was starting to struggle and a roller coaster ensued of biopsies, unsure medical staff on what was causing this and me becoming more and more exhausted by regular trips to hospital for tests and hanging on for what was coming next. The kidney quite miraculously stabilised however damage was already done to the renal tissue by the inflammatory response being triggered and the diagnosis was antibody mediated rejection.

The kidney hung in there for another three and a half years which allowed me to truly explore my own humanity, to look my fears right in the face and trust that all would be well. I began to understand that healing happens in many forms. There are so many layers and aspects to move through. These years saw me dive much deeper into my yoga practice including meditations and mantras and a willingness to heal my wounds from the past. This decline in kidney function to circa 16% prompted me to follow my heart and I stepped away fully from corporate life.

I resigned and had nothing but a chorus of support from colleagues at work. I knew I was doing the right thing. It was time to fully commit to my path and so I focussed fully now on Wholly Aligned, on helping people in their own unique healing journey through yoga and nutrition. It was humbling to continue to be of service to others and lessened the need for me to feel overwhelmed by my own health challenges. I could still flourish. I marvelled at the resilience of my body.

I visited my cousin in California a few times during these years who is very interested in health and spirituality. I was always exploring options and fascinating practitioners who had a far more holistic view of health and wellbeing than the allopathic doctors at home. I learned more and more how to help myself thrive so I could facilitate this for others. The exploration never ends. I came across a naturopathic doctor in America when my transplant kidney had begun to struggle and had a Skype session with her. She herself had gone through kidney illness including transplantation and dialysis so she understood. It was heartening for me to find such a doctor and her advice was safe and practical and helped me feel that I was taking action. I'm sure this helped to keep me well whilst my kidney was hanging in there at 16% function.

In Spring 2016 along came a hurtling train for my chest. That was the exact vision I had so knew its power was going to be intense and so I surrendered and it came. A very bad flu virus with the kidney having dipped down to 10% function blasted into my cells. Kidneys hold strong reserves for our immunity and vital force and I was just so depleted that there was simply nothing in the tank. As the virus settled its way into my body, a referred bacterial infection began to move into my chest and of course all this pushed the kidney into renal failure.

I did not fully comprehend what was happening and this progressed over the course of a week with me wondering each day that I might improve. I did not improve. I could feel life ebbing out of me. But I wasn't scared at all. At the prompting of my sister I spoke to a doctor who advised me to go straight to A&E given my medical history so off I went accompanied by a good friend. I received all the medical care with great humility and knew it was all needed and my body had come to the edge and was days away from expiring. I was admitted into the renal ward and within hours could already feel an improvement. Antibiotics to bring the chest sepsis under control, strong painkillers to relieve the pounding headache, bicarb drips to address the metabolic acidosis that had set in.

And the much needed emergency dialysis to bring all the uraemic toxins in my blood down. I made the decision to opt for home peritoneal dialysis and so an abdominal catheter was fitted. I processed all of this with presence and attention to my experience. As such it was a beautiful surrender and the preceding years of spiritual excavation had prepared me for this and so I was able to navigate it effortlessly. I was in hospital for a week and then back teaching a week after that which was just remarkable given the context of what had occurred.

I adapted to the night-time dialysis which was just totally different from the teenage years of having to go into a hospital ward for daytime treatments. To me this was the ultimate in self-care. I was trained in how to follow a strict aseptic technique and set up the machine and again this has just become part of my current routine. Can I still thrive? Yes! Can I still forge ahead with the even bigger vision I have for myself to inspire others who might be going through life threatening illness? Yes! I know now the power that comes from sharing our stories. There is no value in remaining hidden. Talking more about this lessens the charge that I used to feel as the emotional pain has vastly dissipated. I need to be able to communicate my story without each time reliving the pain. Once I began to reflect on this, I was able to speak more freely about my experiences in a practical way in order to be of value to others.

A useful way of thinking I have also found helpful is to celebrate what does work in your body. The body and mind are incredibly complex and there is so much happening second to second. The more we are able to explore this, the more empowered we are to take action and to take responsibility. Yoga with all its wisdom and exploration of our physical anatomy also helps us explore the subtle anatomy of our being. The chakras you may have heard of, are energy centres that run throughout the body. They represent a way of journeying through our divine experience more fully. For example, if we wish to connect more with the power of our voice and communicating safely to others what we really feel, we might work on a yoga practice that helps to clear energetic debris from the throat chakra. A thyroid imbalance or regular throat infections might be an indication that this energy centre needs some attention.

Yoga is an ancient art. We tread upon a path towards self-realisation. Remember too that the physical side of yoga, namely the yoga poses, is just one element of yoga. The breath is the integral relationship to be harnessed and embraced. The constant breath that pervades our whole life. What is your relationship with your breath?

I also have become increasingly fascinated by the healing potential of yin yoga. There will always be some aspect of the practice you can dive into no matter what your circumstances. When I was adjusting to having an abdominal catheter I was quite trepidatious about what sort of movement would be appropriate for me. Yin yoga provided a perfect medium for me to attend to my body and mind in a gentle way. It also helped me to reconnect with my strength and I felt confident again to start a stronger practice after a few months. Much of western yoga has been very yang for a long time. Intense and dynamic and really quite masculine. There are many benefits of that style of movement however it is important to create harmony and balance in the body and mind and this is where the softer and surrendering style of yin comes in. The poses in yin yoga are passive - meaning there is a dissolution away from muscular contraction as we move towards accessing the deeper muscles and connective tissue, deliberately loading weight into the joints by holding these passive poses for minutes at a time. A big challenge of course is the realm of the mind can get agitated especially if we are not used to this level of moving into stillness and truthfully observing our human experience. Yin yoga holds its roots in Traditional Chinese Medicine so is strongly influenced by Daoism. The poses are intended to open up the energy lines known as the meridians. If you've ever had acupuncture you will be familiar with this concept. Yin yoga is like a personal acupressure session you give yourself.

Through a regular yoga practise, we can then start to delve more into what foods honour our body and why. When we discover that all is energy, perhaps we are more likely to take care over our choices of nourishment. We can then feel the vital force of the food we take into our bodies, for example a loved one making us a bowl of homemade soup full of goodness when we are feeling poorly. The energy of love that has gone into that bowl of food is as meaningful as the ingredients. One of the great memories I have after I was discharged from hospital in 2016 and my friend George coming to visit with his girlfriend. He called to say they were coming over and asked what I would like. He said that if there was something I would really enjoy, I should just ask for it and he would find it.

Accepting kindness can be very healing too. Often we don't wish to be a burden and might say, oh no that's fine. However I said I'd have a think and let him know. So I sat on my sofa feeling into what food I really wanted. And the answer appeared - it was rotisserie chicken! I hadn't been eating much meat at all in recent years however I just had this image and could almost smell the rotisserie chicken. So that was my request to George. They arrived a bit later sweeping in with the most delicious wood fired garlic and lemon organic rotisserie chicken (George knows me well!) with side orders of roasted peppers and red onions.   This was brought to me with such love and consideration I almost cried when I ate it. I listened to my body and what it needed, probably craving protein and iron after having been so unwell. I can still taste those flavours now when I recall it. For my fortieth birthday party a few months later I ordered the very same food for us all to enjoy. That is the power of food and a shared heart-warming moment.

I have come to realise we are all so unique. This is very important to understand when it comes to managing your own health and wellbeing. You are unique and therefore only you know what feels right for your body, for your mind, for your spirit. All aspects of ourselves require nurturing. For me yoga and nutrition are incredibly valuable tools to help me to nurture the whole. What is so remarkable about nutrition as a tool is that it applies to everyone. We all require food to sustain us. If we have not had the fortune of a useful foundation around food as children, it can be very challenging to change patterns as adults. But the old adage of it's never too late to start is true. As my dad says, the body is very forgiving. Our cells will sing back to us when we nourish them well. The body has tremendous capacity to heal and regenerate. But of course we need to believe that is so too. We learn the language of our own body. This takes time to attune to your own intricate vocabulary. What I really felt during those years the transplant kidney began to decline is compassion. Compassion for my own experiences. It was so humbling. To acknowledge what I have been through and also let it go so it does not propel me into poor choices or stuck emotions. I am now over eighteen months on peritoneal dialysis and listed to have a second kidney transplant. My focus is to remain healthy and strong whilst knowing too that is contextual to me. Healthy and strong to me will feel entirely different to healthy and strong in another. There are a number of physiological factors I need to consider due to my kidney dysfunction as the kidneys contribute so much as major organs to our wellness. I have the gift of education and knowledge alongside years of experience that help me to include things in my life to counter the effects of the dialysis treatment. Dialysis gets you by, it is in no way a like for like replacement for the amazing kidneys. It does about 10% of what our kidneys do.

I also am very mindful not to resent the treatment as it is a life support. This is why I say hello to my dialysis machine when I come into my bedroom and set an intention that each treatment is safe and effective. I learned from an early age that resenting the treatment was a sure decline in mental wellbeing and to see it as a gift rather than a hindrance and celebrate too that there are options. How amazing that I received a beautiful kidney from a man who had passed away and how wonderful that the kidney lasted almost two decades, seeing me through my twenties and most of my thirties. I also appreciate where I am now. I have created a life for myself that allows me to rest when I need to and enjoy the moments when I feel energised so I can dance, I can go to the gym, I can go on big walks in nature and drink in the medicine from the trees and the landscape, the fresh air.

And I can share my story with you. And be of service for those who are called to seek me out, whether your health issue is kidney related or you just need some tools to help you relax and breathe more deeply.

There is a saying in shamanism, another area I have dived into in recent years that I just love, 'When you have found your song and you have found your dance, you are home.' Find what makes you sing from within, seek out people who truly see you, share your stories so they don't remain buried in your cells causing disease and upset. We all share the common experience of having a human body, of having thoughts, of breathing. Dive into your human experience and create the circumstances that nourish you. Together we create the beautiful language of wellbeing.

By Ciara Jean Roberts

About the author

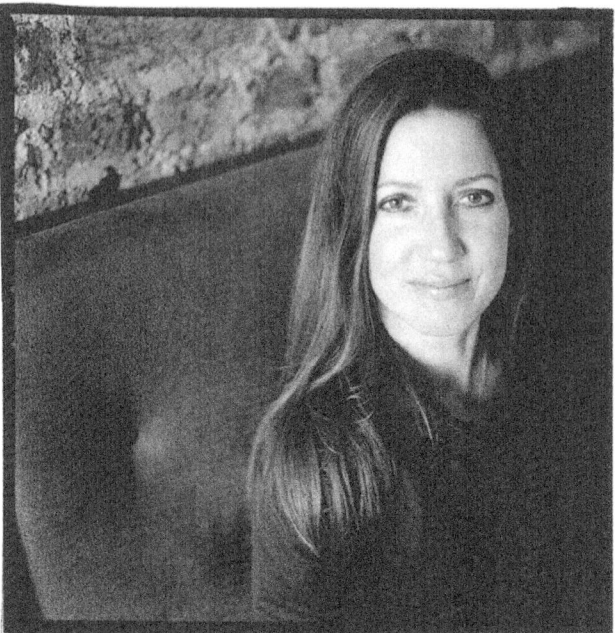

Ciara Jean Roberts is a naturopathic nutritionist, yoga teacher and writer. She has had kidney issues for most of her life. She therefore understands first-hand the importance of empowering yourself with your choices and finding the tools that resonate truthfully with you as the unique person you are in order to feel your best.

Following a hectic career in private banking in London, a change in her health prompted her to listen to her calling to be of service to others and she set up Wholly Aligned, her own endeavour using personalised nutrition and yoga to help people navigate their way to wellness and into alignment in both mind and body. Stepping away form the corporate world, she never looked back.

She has featured in Yoga Magazine, Top Sante and Journal of Kidney Care among many other publications. Her more recent project Harmony Hour, Wholly Aligned is a new YouTube channel bringing uplifting interviews, yoga sequences, music and dance to the community.

She strongly advocates that empowerment comes through taking responsibility for our circumstances and how we can evolve through our experiences with courage, vulnerability and grace.

In more recent years she has been increasingly drawn to shamanic wisdom spending a summer in the Andes in Peru diving more deeply into this ancient wisdom. She completed a Master Apprenticeship in Magic, Medicine and Mysticism with the formidable Peruvian curandero Don Oscar Miro Quesada. She is currently completing her own book detailing her journey. She lives in Crystal Palace, London.

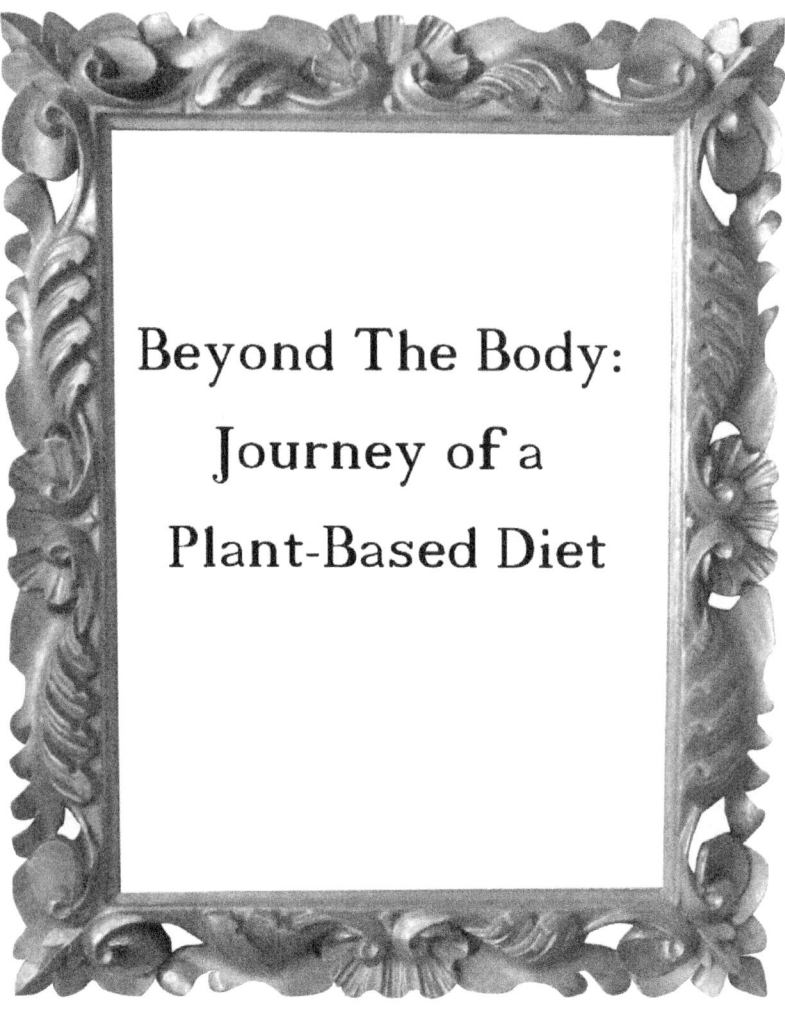

Beyond The Body: Journey of a Plant-Based Diet

Beyond The Body: Journey of a Plant-Based Diet

I want to tell you a little story.

A moment in time, that became the gateway to my plant-based vegan journey. A moment that became my gateway to understanding that a vegan diet was not just 'kale and cucumber'

In 2010 my life was incredibly ordinary. Everything was very mediocre. Not bad, but really not great either. Towards the end of that year I met a guy, a vegan guy.

One weekend on our third date, we went for a walk around a park which led into the town centre where the office building of the company he owned was based. We had grabbed some lunch from the supermarket and were debating where to sit and eat it. He asked if I'd like to come up and see his office as it was on the 12th floor of the building and had a great view over the town. It would be empty and we could sit and eat lunch there.

He was right, the view was amazing.

He took a 'Nakd bar' (equivalent to Larabar in the US) out of his carrier bag and I looked over curiously, since I had already finished all my food! Breaking it in half he held out his hand, with a bemused and slightly quizzical look on his face.

"It's just dates, nuts and cocoa all smooshed up together…it tastes exactly like chocolate", he told me.

"Yeah right" I smiled back.

But I very was curious, and to be honest didn't want to offend since it was only the third date and all! So I took it.

Mind blown. It DID taste exactly like chocolate!

In that precise moment in time, as I sat on a chair on the 12th floor of an empty office block with a guy I barely knew... my entire life changed. In that precise moment I realised that a vegan diet was indeed about more than just kale and cucumber... I was holding the proof in my hand!

I still vividly remember thinking, 'maybe this guy is not so crazy after all!'

At that time veganism was not at all mainstream (I'd even had to ask him to explain to me exactly what it meant!) Vegan food options were not widely available and Nakd bars were pretty much the only type of vegan treat you could buy, and only typically available in health food shops. Plus they were very expensive!

From that moment forward my curiosity got the better of me. I made vegan cakes and cookies that he could eat at every given opportunity. I went and bought a £20 food processor on Amazon so I could make my own chocolate 'smoosh bars'. It wasn't until about nine months later than my 'Including Cake' recipe blog was born, by which time I was now totally immersed in it, following a 99% healthy, wholefood plant-based diet myself and seeing so many shifts in all areas of my life- physically, mentally and spiritually.

In conversations with others, I often refer to myself as an 'accidental vegan', since it had never even been on my radar. Life simply presented me with a guy, who happened to offer me a piece of chocolate Nakd bar one day and in doing so turned my world around,

---

Over the last six years since that moment, I have grown and evolved so deeply and I attribute so much of this to shifting to a plant-based wholefood diet. I often talk about nutrition being the gateway to our optimal self, because it literally creates the foundation for the journey, it provides us with the building blocks at a cellular level.

Of course I appreciate there are many of interpretations of a 'healthy diet' but my focus here is specifically my experience of the benefits of a plant-based diet and not only my experiences, but those of so many clients, colleagues and friends around the world who have shared with me their incredible shifts too.

Let's first consider some of the fundamental benefits of a plant-based diet in relation to our physical wellbeing.

In removing the animal products we create a more alkaline environment, which is often referred to as the 'healing diet'. One of the things I personally noticed almost immediately when I'd made the shift was that the speed of muscle recovery after heavy gym training was significantly improved, there was less inflammation in my body and so less muscle soreness.

Reduction in inflammation across the body, enables the muscles to work more efficiently with less energy expenditure- giving us more energy to use elsewhere.

That is also referred to as 'high net gain nutrition', where we are spending a small amount of digestive energy for a big nutritional return.

We are in the age of discoveries, yet so many people still suffer an energy crisis - they are constantly fatigued, susceptible to tension and anxiety, disease and depression. People seem to vary between complete disregard for what they eat and a fanatical obsession with proteins, vitamins, minerals and calories. As a society we have disregarded going back to basics. Back to abundant plant-based wholefoods.

We don't even have to eat a lot of food to be well nourished, in fact it's the nutritional density that matters, that is the ratio between the amount of calories in a given food to its nutritional value- vitamins, minerals, phytochemicals and antioxidants. Brightly and intensely coloured fruits and veg are highest in antioxidants. We want to consume as much of each nutrient relative to the amount of calories. If we base our diets on the nutrient dense plant-based wholefoods, we'll be sure of getting the highest level of nutrition in.

Another noticeable sign very early on in my transition, was my increased energy and reduced need for sleep. I'd literally be bouncing out of bed early in the morning, something that had never happened before! When we eat alkaline foods overall nutritional stress goes down which also reduces the levels of cortisol- the stress hormone, enabling higher quality sleep.

It was experiencing positive physical changes like this, that gave me huge motivation to continue the exploration.

Shifting across to a mind-body viewpoint, a wholefood plant-based diet, by its very nature means that we are eating closer to the Source. The more refined and processed the foods we eat, the more we are travelling away from the original source, and so arguably the energy from the 'life source' is reduced. This effect is even more dramatically enhanced when we shift to a more 'raw vegan' diet also known as a 'high vibrational' or 'living food' diet.

A high vibrational diet is described as a diet consists of foods that are 'alive' and that positively benefit the person, as well as the planet as a whole. High vibration means having more light, and thus less density. Plants exemplify this by photosynthesizing light into energy.

Spiritual nutrition also ties in with the idea of eating closer to source. Originating in Buddhist and Hindu communities is the idea of 'Ahimsa', where the wellbeing of everything that is related to the food itself is considered. It is thought that a more plant-based diet offers access to the higher self. Mahatma Gandhi was a great exponent of ahimsa, saying, "The way to truth lies through ahimsa."

Recently, I spent some time living with a number of different spiritual communities around the world, all of which followed a plant-based vegetarian or vegan lifestyle. It was fascinating to observe the ways in which their diet and lifestyle was so interconnected.

In speaking with a resident at one of the centres I stayed at, he talked of a deep sense of wellbeing and a knowledge that "every day I am living and eating with a purpose that extends beyond myself." I found myself nodding and realising that for me too, there is so much truth in that statement.

Prior to switching to a plant-based wholefood diet, I had not considered myself a particularly spiritual person, yet now these were the people I was drawn to and most resonated with. I also found that the ethical side and 'wider view' of a vegan lifestyle was slowly beginning to catch up with me, and link arms with the nutritional standpoint that had first caught my attention and led me down the road in the beginning.

As my fascination with a plant based-diet grew, I found myself more and more drawn into conversations with others who had found themselves on a similar path, often triggered by very different start points.

I began a series of interviews as a platform for sharing the stories of those who have created powerful transformation in their lives through plant-based nutrition as the gateway to change. Nutrition is a powerful catalyst... but, as I soon discovered, it is just the beginning. It creates a threshold to allow you to step more powerfully into your own story of wellness in ways you would never have thought possible.

The first person I interviewed was a guy I met whilst in Portugal. He'd turned his entire life on its head, leaving the UK and his well paid building company to set up an off-grid community and retreat centre in the Portuguese mountains.

I was fascinated as to what triggered this. He told me that it was through years of battling debilitating Crohn's disease that at times almost killed him and according to the medical profession was 'incurable', but was then totally cured by switching to a plant-based whole food diet as a last resort. What began as a '30-day plant-based challenge' following advice from a trusted friend turned into his life's purpose.

What is fascinating is that he also realised that after about six months of being fully plant-based, the asthma that had plagued him his entire life, with attacks often landing him in hospital, had totally disappeared.

He told me; "My whole life has done 180 degree shift, most of my friends back home don't know me any more. I am a better version of myself. After the initial 30-days I wanted more, what else could I do? The next thing was yoga and meditation, what could I do with my body and mind? I had been a typical gym lad, wanting to build big bulky muscle, and so yoga could not have been a bigger shift for me. I began questioning everything else in my life. I went with what felt right for me in my heart".

Whilst the stories of those I interviewed could not have been more different, there were some fascinating patterns that quickly began to emerge.

Another lady, now the creator of a healthy food and lifestyle magazine, told me; "You start on the journey with what you're eating but then your mind opens up and you find your intuition becomes more empowered as your nutrition improves."

Another interview alludes to this same sense of mind-body shift;

"Two weeks after going vegan the eczema that had plagued me for years just disappeared. The fact that I saw the physical benefit straightaway gave me the motivation to continue. After a few months had past I noticed I had not had a single depressive episode or self-harmed. I would say that through a vegan diet I am completely cured of depression. I feel content and grounded in myself."

In all my conversations, the sense of 'expansion' was very apparent and also very much part of my own story.

Once we stop and question something so integral such as diet, something that is so deeply conditioned to be perceived a certain way in our society, and we realise there are other solutions... it creates a cascade of questioning. The better we feel the more we question and the more in tune we become with our inner knowing.

Very soon another question began to rise within me. Does a plant-based diet increase your innate creativity?

This had been something I had been feeling for some time. When I made the shift to a plant-based wholefood diet, my own creativity sky rocketed. I had always been a creative person in the traditional 'arty' sense, but now coupled with the questioning mentality, my creativity and curiosity knew no bounds.

I also had a sense that creativity and a sense of wellbeing were inextricably and powerfully linked. Indeed, a quick search on-line brings up numerous articles and research literature on how being more creative improves our mental and physical health. This deeper approach to well-being is often described as "eudaimonic well-being" and focuses on living life in a full and deeply satisfying way.

Creativity is fundamental to the experience of being human.

The deep connection between creativity and meaning was noted long ago by the creativity researcher Frank X. Barron. Through his pioneering research on some of the most creative people of his generation, Barron came to realize that creative people have the remarkable capacity to become intimate with themselves. According to psychologist Ruth Richards, they "dare to look within, even at one's irrational and less conscious material, including one's 'shadow' materials". Richards refers to this capacity as "courageous openness".

As Richards puts it, "A creative style of living, coping with difficulties and weaving possibilities, can not only produce useful accomplishments for self and world but can offer the creator new resilience, perspective, aliveness in the moment, joy, and purpose in life."

In the words of Brene Brown; "Creativity is the way I share my soul with the world." I see creativity as giving yourself permission to see things differently. Tilting your perspective, maybe mere millimeters, to create the world anew and shine a light into previously undiscovered corners.

For me the shift is primarily two-fold; Once we go against the norms and think outside the box in terms of what we put on our plates, it opens up space to question the world beyond the confines of society's expectations and gives us courage to step into our authentic truth in so many other ways. Alongside this, the nourishment for our body through eating closer to source creates a 'lightness', an increased energy at a cellular level and something of a spiritual connection within, although I didn't realise this initially and still find it hard to put into words today.

I decided to reach out to see if others shared my thoughts and feelings around a plant-based diet and innate creativity. I put this question out to various plant-based communities: *"Do you feel as though your creativity, spirituality or personal development has increased significantly since switching to a plant-based vegan diet?"* I received an overwhelming majority of 'Yes's to my poll, approx 70%. Some beautiful comments were shared which strongly reinforced for me this powerful dietary link and mindset catalyst.

Here are some of the words that were shared:

"Yes! absolutely it has! I have been vegan just over a year and it has had a positive impact on all areas of my life. I think on a deeper level, I am more connected to the earth and I am more peaceful. I have had more creative ideas and energy to make them a reality."

"I went vegetarian the beginning of last year and have gone vegan this month, I have to say my creativity has increased! I am drawing and painting again, something I haven't done in a long time. Also in the way I am being creative in my wardrobe and dressing more how I want too!"

"I am much more creative since going vegan. I'm not sure if it has to do with nutrition as much as living a more authentic and value based lifestyle. It has pushed me out of the dissatisfied way I had been living. I'm also more fearless, I try new things all the time. "

"A vegetarian for 30 years, I then embraced a raw vegan lifestyle about 3 years ago which totally changed me. I suddenly felt connected with the earth, with nature, with life in a way I never had before. Alive, creative, excited.... It was transformative! 3 years down the line I don't eat a wholly raw diet any more, I eat a mostly vegan diet (eggs from my pet ducks when they're laying) but with a high proportion of raw because when you eat raw foods you really feel the life-force, the energy, of those foods going into your body and it's wonderful."

"I can certainly relate to this. I've metamorphosed from a bored meal provider into an enthusiastic, energetic and lovable (well my family believe so) server of wholesome foods. One's creative energies seem to open up in so many areas of one's life."

"Yes, not only in cooking but other ways too. I always have been the type to look outside the box anyway, but this perspective on life has changed the way I look at things even more."

It's not just feedback on social media that align with this way of thinking. I dug a little deeper and found various articles also alluding to this sense of creativity and connectedness. Back in 2008 Steve Pavlina wrote a long article focussed on 'diet and energy'. It document's the authors thoughts around his shift to a raw vegan diet. He states, the most significant and biggest change was definitely increased creative output.

"I feel more creatively inspired than ever, so I've been doing more creative work than I used to, shifting between blogging, speaking, journaling, business planning, concocting raw food dishes, and other outlets. I now feel very uncomfortable if I go more than a couple days without creating new material. It's like I'm overly aroused with creative energy and feel compelled to express it." I was also fascinated by the question he asked in the article; "Are you resisting a more energetic state of being?

"If you improve your diet and then feel much more energetic (physically, mentally, emotionally, and spiritually), how will you channel all that extra energy? Where will you direct it? How will you use it to fuel greater creative output? I think those questions need to be addressed before you're ready to make the shift. Otherwise it's too easy to fall back into your old comfort zone."

This is fascinating to me, and something I had never before considered in that light. When I work with coaching clients or speak with friends who are struggling with aspects of their nutritional journey, or indeed any aspect of stepping up and changing their life for the better, the idea that clinging to our comfort zone, or as Steve put's it 'resisting a more energetic state of being' begins to make a lot of sense. Whilst we all, no doubt, want to achieve a state of optimal well-being, we also need to be ready for it. No more hiding behind the stories we tell ourselves that keep us playing small. I believe there is a powerful truth in the 'knowing'. That when you know more; when you have experienced it in the heart of your being, then there is no 'un-knowing'. Exploring Veganism and a plant-based diet goes beyond the body and expands the mind in so many dimensions, and a mind expanded cannot return to its old dimensions.

By Jo Hodson

About the author

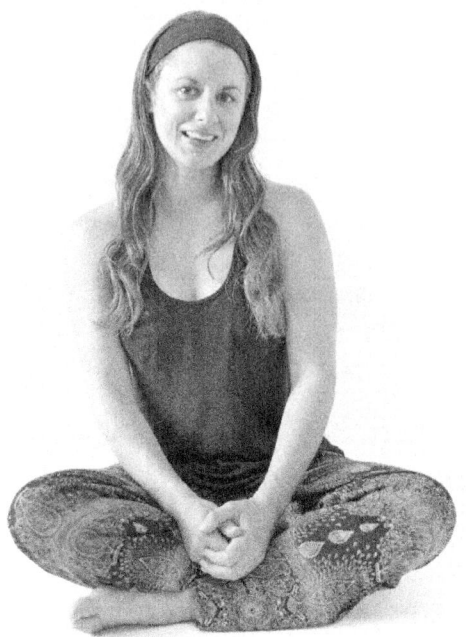

Jo is the health & mindset coach behind the website Including Cake. Her passion was born from a personal journey of nutrition being a gateway for creativity and a deeper connection with her innate sense of self and wellbeing.

You can find more about Jo's work and explore plenty of creative plant-based recipes and mindset motivation over at includingcake.com

Social media links:

https://www.facebook.com/includingcake

https://www.instagram.com/johodson

https://twitter.com/IncludingCake

Kizzi's Health and Well-Being

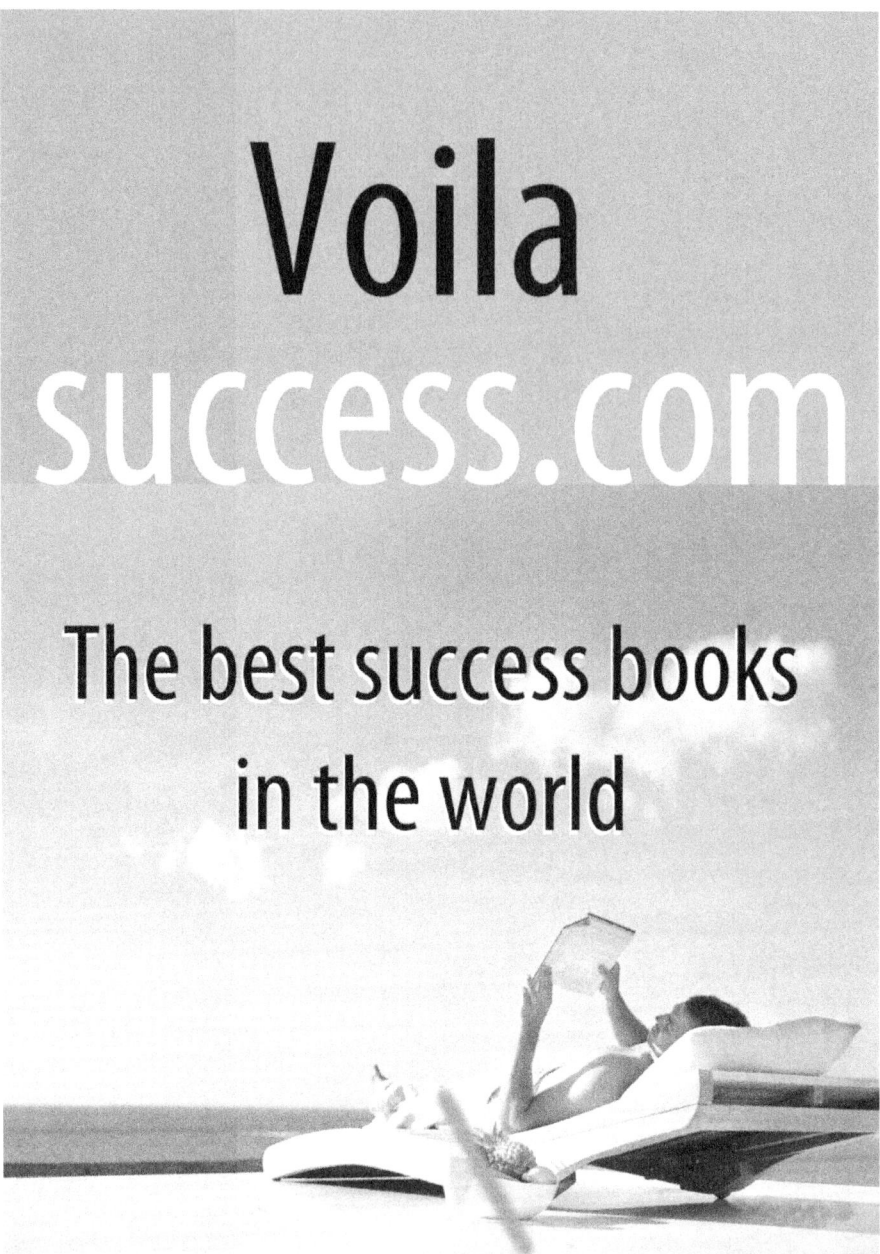
Kizzi's Health and Well-Being

THIRD EDITION
THE BOOK OF SUCCESS

EDITED BY KIZZI NKWOCHA

Written by the some of the world's greatest NLP, lifestyle and motivation experts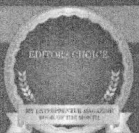

YOUR GUIDE TO THE PROGRESSIVE REALIZATION OF A WORTHY IDEAL

SPONSORED BY MY ENTREPRENEUR MAGAZINE

Kizzi's Health and Well-Being

Kizzi's Health and Well-Being

Printed by Amazon Italia Logistica S.r.l.
Torrazza Piemonte (TO), Italy